Lessons Learned:
Stories from Women in
Medical Management

edited by
Deborah M. Shlian, MD, MBA

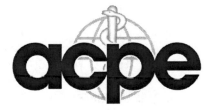

Pam,

Great book by
great women! :)

Best,
Hoda

acpe

American College of Physician Executives
400 North Ashley Drive, Suite 400
Tampa, Florida 33602
800-562-8088 • 813-287-2000

ISBN: 978-0-924674-45-7

Library of Congress Card Number: 2012950805

Printed in the United States of America by Lightning Source

FOREWORD

Are we there yet?

In 1995, the American College of Physician Executives (ACPE) published the first monograph in which 17 women physician executives addressed their careers, both in medicine and management. At that time, most of the contributors were primary care physicians in middle management or just beginning to transition from clinical medicine to management roles.

Seventeen years later, there have been substantial changes in medicine, not the least of which is the sheer numbers of women entering medical schools and the wider variety of choices they have in terms of specialties and career paths. Medical management has become a more mature profession and many health care organizations recognize the benefits of having physicians in leadership positions.

In this current version of *Women in Medicine and Management*, 24 women physician executives tell their personal stories: how they chose medicine, why and how they moved into leadership roles, the value of formal management degrees, and how they balance work and personal life. The majority of this group are in senior management. They are diverse demographically, geographically, and specialty-wise. They represent virtually every area of health-care: government, academia, hospitals, provider groups, managed care, the pharmaceutical industry and consulting. A few are entrepreneurs, having started and run their own companies.

While it's true that for the most part, these women would answer the question, *"Are we there yet?"* with a *"Yes,"* they are also aware that they still represent a small percentage of the potential leadership pool among women physicians. And that needs to change.

The Overview section of this monograph explores some of reasons for the so-called "glass ceiling" (or perhaps better called "gauze ceiling") specific to female physicians aspiring to senior executive positions. One of these is the lack of mentors - especially women to women. As President-elect of the American Medical Women's Association (AMWA), I believe that it is fundamentally important for women to occupy as many positions of power as possible within the health care system, not only because we will soon make up the majority of physicians, but because we bring vast talent and energy combined with our own unique perspectives to the table. One of my personal goals is to help create more mentoring opportunities for women physicians throughout their careers, from undergraduate and medical school to physician leader.

In my opinion, there's a sweet spot in heaven for women who smooth the way for other women. Each time one woman is elevated because another woman helped her move up, all women are elevated. Women working together as a group are stronger than the sum of individual efforts. An essential key to women's advancement is women supporting each other through mentoring, coaching, and collaboration. I assume most, if not all of you reading this, are already members of ACPE, but I encourage you to join AMWA as well. Involvement in AMWA gives the opportunity to contribute to the progress of not only women physicians but the opportunity to advance women's health care issues and the condition of women globally.

It is essential to appreciate the barriers women still face as they strive for leadership roles in medicine and to learn from each other's experiences, both successes and challenges. The stories of the women profiled in these pages can be a guide, not only for students and young physicians at the beginning of their careers who are considering becoming leaders in health care, but also for those physicians who may be in mid career or even beyond who are interested in leadership and management options.

If we're not there yet, then we're definitely on our way!

Bonnie C. Hamilton, MD, FAAP
President-elect American Medical Women's Association, 2012-13
Fairfield, California
bonnie.hamilton@sbcglobal.net

CONTENTS

PROVIDER GROUPS

MANAGED CARE (FOR PROFIT AND NOT-FOR-PROFIT)

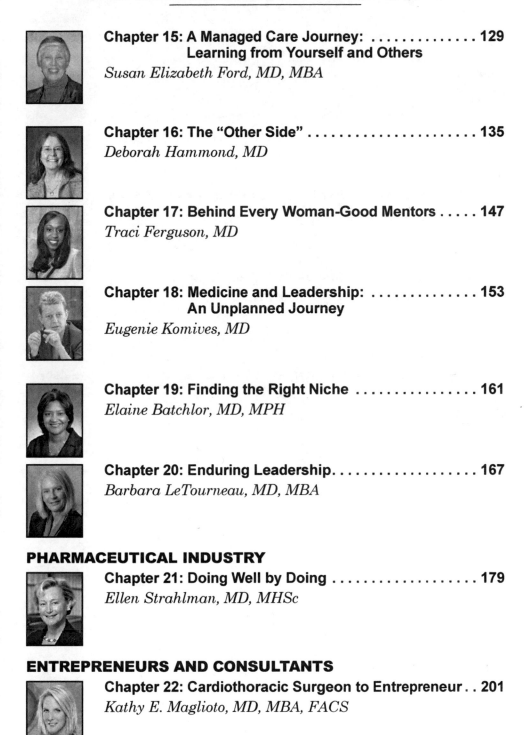

CHAPTER ONE

An Overview

"How did you get into medical management?" is a question that even in 2012 sometimes carries the same implications as, "What is a nice girl like you doing in a place like this?"

The sense that medical administration is not an appropriate career goal for a woman physician was just beginning to change with the publication of the first version of "Women in Medicine and Management" in 1995. At that time women represented about 19 percent of all American physicians. That was a jump from just under 8 percent in 1970. Between 1980 and 2009, the number of female physicians increased 430 percent, so by 2009, 30 percent of practicing physicians in the United States were women[1].

In terms of specialties, there have been significant shifts here as well. Only 7 specialties had more than 1000 female physicians in 1970, whereas 25 specialties had more than 1000 female physicians by 2006[1]. Although 60 percent of women physicians are still more prominent in primary care specialties such as family medicine, internal medicine, pediatrics, and obstetrics/gynecology as well as psychiatry and anesthesiology, younger graduates today are choosing residencies in virtually every specialty including cardiothoracic and neurosurgery (Table 1)

According to 2011 AMA statistics, 54 percent of female physicians were under age 45[1]. In 2011, almost half of all medical students were female (Table 2). With the publication of this 2012 update, there are as many as 60 percent

Table 1. Residency Applicants of U.S Medical Schools by Specialty and Sex, 2011

The table below contains the numbers of U.S. medical school graduate residency applicants by gender, and the average number of applications individuals of that gender supplied to programs of the specialty in question. Please e-mail us at facts@aamc.org if you need further assistance or have additional inquiries.

U.S. Medical School Graduate ERAS Users by Specialty and Sex, 2011	Women		Men	
	Applicants	Avg number of Applications	Applicants	Avg number of Applications
Anesthesiology	592	27.8	1,135	29.0
Child Neurology (Neurology)	1	1.0	0	0.0
Dermatology	403	58.5	260	51.0
Emergency Medicine	665	31.0	1,214	31.6
Emergency Medicine/Family Medicine	9	1.8	15	1.5
Family Medicine	1,180	16.6	1,107	17.1
Internal Medicine	3,287	20.8	4,364	20.3
Internal Medicine/Dermatology	73	4.2	51	4.0
Internal Medicine/Emergency Medicine	30	5.2	55	5.3
Internal Medicine/Family Practice	12	1.3	12	1.6
Internal Medicine/Medical Genetics	1	3.0	6	1.7
Internal Medicine/Neurology	3	1.3	3	1.0
Internal Medicine/Pediatrics	269	18.8	186	17.6
Internal Medicine/Preventive Medicine	26	1.5	18	1.9
Internal Medicine/Psychiatry	34	3.2	55	3.3
Neurological Surgery	71	41.8	225	42.2
Neurology	245	22.5	293	19.7
Nuclear Medicine	14	4.7	38	3.6
Obstetrics and Gynecology	938	32.2	228	31.0
Orthopaedic Surgery	171	56.0	903	57.1
Otolaryngology	154	49.3	281	44.4
Pathology-Anatomic and Clinical	253	18.9	287	18.8
Pediatrics	1,674	20.9	632	18.9
Pediatrics/Emergency Medicine	16	2.4	13	2.5
Pediatrics/Medical Genetics	26	2.7	30	2.6
Pediatrics/Physical Medicine and Rehabilitation	11	2.6	5	1.4
Pediatrics/Psychiatry/Child and Adolescent Psychiatry	33	5.7	15	6.3
Physical Medicine and Rehabilitation	148	20.2	259	15.2
Plastic Surgery	71	15.8	144	14.8
Plastic Surgery-Integrated	77	26.1	158	24.4
Preventive Medicine	56	2.9	52	4.7
Psychiatry	518	20.6	480	19.9
Psychiatry/Family Practice	18	3.3	17	3.6
Psychiatry/Neurology	21	1.5	37	1.7
Radiation Oncology	68	41.3	217	40.2
Radiology-Diagnostic	388	42.4	993	44.8
Surgery-General	967	30.8	1,733	26.0
Thoracic Surgery-Integrated	19	6.2	69	7.1
Transitional Year	1,275	8.2	2,018	9.9
Urology	82	49.1	225	47.3
Vascular Surgery-Integrated	45	13.0	77	7.6

Source: AAMC ERAS DW, as of 9/29/2011.

Table 2. Medical Students Enrolled by Year and Gender

MEDICAL STUDENTS, SELECTED YEARS, 1965–2010

Academic Year	APPLICANTS Total	Women	Women as % of Total	ACCEPTED APPLICANTS Total	Women	Women as % of Total	MATRICULANTS Total	Women	Women as % of Total	FIRST-YEAR ENROLLMENT* Total	Women	Women as % of Total	TOTAL ENROLLMENT* Total	Women	Women as % of Total	GRADUATES Total	Women	Women as % of Total
1965–66	18,703	1,676	9.0%	9,012	799	8.9%	8,554	799	9.3%	8,759	731@	8.3%	32,835	2,589	7.9%	7,574	524	6.9%
1970–71	24,987	2,734	10.9%	11,500	1,297	11.3%	11,169	1,228	11.0%	11,348	1,256	11.1%	40,487	3,894	9.6%	8,974	827	9.2%
1975–76†	42,282	9,590	22.7%	15,360	3,642	23.7%	14,897	3,511	23.6%	15,295	3,647	23.8%	55,818	11,417	20.5%	13,634	2,212	16.2%
1980–81	36,083	10,657	29.5%	17,141	4,948	28.9%	16,587	4,757	28.7%	17,186	4,966	28.9%	65,189‡	17,248	26.5%	15,632	3,898	24.9%
1985–86	32,885	11,563	35.1%	17,225	5,857	34.0%	16,268	5,520	33.9%	16,963	5,800	34.2%	66,585	21,650	32.5%	16,117	4,957	30.8%
1990–91	29,241	11,783	40.3%	17,206	6,656	38.7%	15,998	6,153	38.5%	16,876	6,550	38.8%	65,163	24,286	37.3%	15,427	5,553	36.0%
1991–92	33,297	13,699	41.1%	17,435	6,943	39.8%	16,211	6,433	39.7%	17,071	6,804	39.9%	65,602	24,962	38.1%	15,356	5,543	36.1%
1992–93	37,402	15,618	41.8%	17,465	7,257	41.6%	16,289	6,772	41.6%	17,097	7,158	41.9%	65,606	25,754	39.3%	15,474	5,890	38.1%
1993–94	42,806	17,957	41.9%	17,361	7,288	42.0%	16,307	6,851	42.0%	17,121	7,230	42.2%	66,202	26,589	40.2%	15,504	5,895	38.0%
1994–95	45,360	18,967	41.8%	17,318	7,265	41.9%	16,287	6,819	41.9%	17,085	7,212	42.2%	66,815	27,364	41.0%	15,883	6,228	39.2%
1995–96	46,586	19,773	42.5%	17,356	7,437	42.8%	16,252	6,941	42.7%	17,058	7,363	43.2%	66,947	27,925	41.7%	15,895	6,501	40.9%
1996–97	46,965	20,028	42.6%	17,385	7,439	42.8%	16,201	6,918	42.7%	16,935	7,271	42.9%	66,913	28,157	42.1%	15,894	6,595	41.5%
1997–98	43,016	18,271	42.5%	17,312	7,484	43.2%	16,164	6,994	43.3%	16,867	7,333	43.5%	69,089	29,205	42.3%	15,972	6,656	41.7%
1998–99	40,996	17,785	43.4%	17,373	7,685	44.2%	16,170	7,162	44.3%	16,790**	7,450**	44.4%	69,297	29,680	42.8%	16,006	6,792	42.4%
1999–00	38,443	17,395	45.2%	17,421	7,966	45.7%	16,221	7,412	45.7%	16,856^	450^	45.7%	69,303	30,179	43.5%	15,716	6,675	42.5%
2000–01	37,088	17,273	46.6%	17,535	8,027	45.8%	16,301	7,472	45.8%	16,699	7,659	45.9%	69,413	30,739	44.3%	15,794	6,824	43.2%
2001–02	34,860	16,718	48.0%	17,454	8,294	47.5%	16,365	7,784	47.6%	16,875	8,039	47.6%	69,518	31,492	45.3%	15,676	6,923	44.2%
2002–03	33,624	16,556	49.2%	17,592	8,631	49.1%	16,488	8,113	49.2%	16,953	8,311	49.0%	69,930	32,452	46.4%	15,532	7,029	45.3%
2003–04	34,791	17,672	50.8%	17,542	8,732	49.8%	16,541	8,212	49.6%	17,035	8,470	49.7%	70,313	33,331	47.4%	15,829	7,261	45.9%
2004–05	35,735	18,018	50.4%	17,662	8,768	49.6%	16,648	8,235	49.5%	17,059	8,433	49.4%	71,028	34,261	48.2%	15,760	7,412	47.0%
2005–06	37,372	18,625	49.8%	17,986	8,765	48.7%	17,003	8,239	48.5%	17,376	8,416	48.4%	72,000	34,929	48.5%	15,927	7,748	48.6%
2006–07	39,108	19,293	49.3%	18,418	8,943	48.6%	17,361	8,438	48.6%	17,826	8,678	48.7%	73,111	35,470	48.5%	16,140	7,925	49.1%
2007–08	42,315	20,735	49.0%	18,858	9,107	48.3%	17,759	8,582	48.3%	18,287	8,863	48.5%	74,525	36,005	48.3%	16,169	7,969	49.3%
2008–09	42,231	20,360	48.2%	19,135	9,181	48.0%	18,036	8,614	47.8%	18,370	8,798	47.9%	76,202	36,533	47.9%	16,467	8,036	48.8%
2009–10	42,269	20,252	47.9%	19,332	9,264	47.9%	18,390	8,817	47.9%	18,853	9,109	48.3%	77,722	37,129	47.8%	16,818	8,127	48.3%

Notes

For 1995–96 to present, the applicant and matriculant data are derived from AAMC Data Warehouse (DW): Applicant Matriculant File, updated as of 1/4/2010.

Starting with 2000–01, the First-Year Enrollment data are from the Student Records System (SRS)

Starting with 1992–93, the Total Enrollment and Graduates data are from the DW: Student section and SRS; Total Enrollment is reported as of October 31 of the academic year.

Total active enrollments for 1998–99 forward are derived from DW: Student section on 10/19/2009. Graduates for 1995–1996 forward are derived from DW Student section on 7/8/2010.

Differences in Total Enrollment between years may not be statistically significant. Data starting in 1992–93 are biased slightly toward undercounting, as some cases (less than 1%) were necessarily excluded due to insufficient enrollment status information.

@ 1965–66 First-Year Enrollment count of women is taken from the *Journal of Medical Education*, February 1973, p.188

† 1975–76 Totals include less than one percent for whom gender information was not available.

‡ 1980–81 Total Enrollment count includes 55 students for whom gender information was not available.

* First-Year Enrollment figures include new entrants and those repeating the initial year.

** 1998–99 First-Year Enrollment counts are taken from the *Journal of Medical Education*. September 1999, p.891.

^ 1999–00 First-Year Enrollment Total is derived from LCME Part II, 1997–98, 1998–99, and 1999–00. Gender information is not available.

female students enrolled in a number of medical school classes across the country. While the progress of women doctors has been sometimes a slow, albeit continuing journey, it may not be long before women dominate medicine.

These trends are creating a quiet gender revolution—one that brings new opportunities and tensions. Within the broader context of the evolving role of women in American society, women physicians continue to explore new career paths—paths that include both clinical medicine and medical management.

Power and Promotion

The good news is that women have been entering medicine in increasing numbers for more than three decades. The not so good news is that women are still underrepresented and underutilized in positions of power—especially at the most senior levels. Unfortunately fifty years after the so-called "sexual revolution", there is a relative paucity of women in positions of power in every single sector across this nation. Speaking at a White House conference on urban economic development, Barnard College president Debora Spar stated: "We have fallen into what I call the 16 percent ghetto, which is that if you look at any sector, be it aerospace, engineering, Hollywood films, higher education, or Fortune 500 leading positions, women max out at roughly 16 percent. That is a crime, and it is a waste of incredible talent."[2] A similar situation exists for women in politics. At a mere 16.8 percent of House membership, women's representation in the United States' national legislature last year ranked 78th in the world, tied with Turkmenistan, according to statistics compiled by the Inter-Parliamentary Union.[3]

In reviewing the latest figures on women physicians, it appears that medicine mirrors those statistics. According to the AMA, female physicians represent about 20 percent of physicians in administration (a jump from only 1 percent self-identified as administrators in 2006), but the data do not specify the level at which these women physicians manage[1].

Academia

Studies of women in academic medicine uniformly show that although the numbers have definitely increased since 1995, (the latest statistics indicate that female physicians represent 27.4 percent of physicians in medical teaching and 22.3 percent in research[1]), disparities still persist in their advancement[4-8]. In one recent study, the number of women who advanced to the ranks of associate and full professor was significantly lower than expected (only 16 percent of MD faculty at the full professor rank are female). This is true for both tenured and non-tenured tracks even after adjustment for the department (Table 3). Instead, women continue to cluster in characteristically untenured faculty positions, largely in traditionally "nurturing" specialties, and primarily in administrative posts dealing exclusively with student and minority affairs. For example, out of 137 deans of US medical schools today, only 13 are women (Table 4)

Since academic productivity is cited as the primary reason for the gender gap, Darcy Reed and colleagues compared publication records, academic promotion and leadership appointments of women and men academic physicians at the Mayo Clinic over the span of their entire careers using a longitudinal cohort design[9]. While Mayo is admittedly an untenured system unlike the typical tenured academic model, the study revealed that although the academic productivity of women lagged behind men in the early and middle stages of careers, publication rates were similar between genders in the later stage of academic careers. The authors concluded that academic productivity in mid-career may not be an appropriate measure of leadership skills for women, stating that: "a paucity of qualified women in leadership positions both deprives organizations of the unique skills and perspectives women bring to such roles."

In 2011, after reviewing the literature and finding little information as to why women physicians chose academia, Nicole Borges, PhD and her colleagues did their own study[10]. Not surprising, the authors discovered that the decision is influenced by the environment in which one trains and the various mentors medical students and residents meet along the way. Many women physicians entering academic medicine do so after or during fellowship, which is when they are exposed to this option. Most who responded to Borges' survey stated that an interest in teaching was the primary reason for their choice. For others, academic medicine was described as "a serendipitous or circumstantial choice" rather than a planned one.

Hospitals

Women (physicians and non-physicians) are likewise underrepresented at the highest levels of hospital administration, despite the fact that today women comprise at least 78 percent of the health care industry's workforce and are the largest consumers of health care. A 2005 study of the Solucient 100 top hospitals considered to be the highest quality and leading institutions revealed that of the 474 chief administrators, only 24 percent were women[11]. One third of these hospitals employed no female chief administrators, while another one third employed only one female chief administrator. Female chief administrators were more likely to be a CIO (chief information officer) or CHR

Table 3. Distribution of U.S. Medical School Faculty by Gender and Rank

Rank/Tenure Status	Asian Male	Asian Female	Black Male	Black Female	Native American/Alaskan Male	Native American/Alaskan Female	Native Hawaiian/OPI Male	Native Hawaiian/OPI Female	White Male	White Female	Other Race Male	Other Race Female	Unknown Race Male	Unknown Race Female	Multiple Races Male	Multiple Races Female
Professor																
Tenured	1,210	277	175	55	5	1	3	1	12,090	2,641	18	3	440	132	167	31
On Track	140	41	19	9	1	0	0	0	1,577	414	0	0	139	29	25	6
Not on Track	579	208	93	43	1	3	4	1	5,622	1,515	19	2	414	109	126	33
Not Available	101	30	33	7	1	0	0	0	1,192	225	1	0	221	51	13	2
Missing	99	40	8	5	1	0	0	0	647	189	1	1	111	25	15	2
Subtotal	2,129	596	328	119	9	4	7	2	21,128	4,984	39	6	1,325	346	346	74
Associate Professor																
Tenured	536	182	75	54	6	2	3	0	3,118	1,158	9	5	202	91	92	29
On Track	490	205	57	33	1	1	3	0	2,320	1,160	12	1	263	128	61	33
Not on Track	1,132	563	240	178	9	5	11	2	6,676	3,322	32	14	720	357	243	127
Not Available	107	50	36	32	0	1	0	0	817	323	2	0	231	121	14	4
Missing	165	100	16	17	1	1	1	0	677	351	7	5	169	97	38	23
Subtotal	2,430	1,100	424	314	17	10	18	2	13,608	6,314	62	25	1,585	794	448	216
Assistant Professor																
Tenured	8	6	3	1	0	0	0	0	54	25	0	0	22	9	2	0
On Track	1,364	798	189	266	18	6	18	9	4,197	2,830	31	26	1,687	1,103	195	131
Not on Track	3,230	2,408	671	855	49	35	52	40	11,729	8,122	84	73	3,720	3,301	502	371
Not Available	241	195	58	72	2	2	1	2	1,281	785	10	4	632	433	34	15
Missing	380	299	74	86	3	3	3	3	1,160	859	4	3	853	662	43	37
Subtotal	5,223	3,706	995	1,280	72	45	74	54	18,421	12,621	129	106	6,914	5,508	776	554
Instructor																
Tenured	1	0	0	0	0	0	0	0	2	1	0	0	3	1	0	0
On Track	56	57	15	31	3	3	1	1	282	383	2	14	209	485	4	5
Not on Track	722	611	118	198	11	8	8	10	2,149	2,369	8	0	1,714	2,064	76	63
Not Available	22	26	8	26	1	0	0	0	141	133	0	0	215	257	2	0
Missing	64	74	14	25	2	2	1	1	214	217	0	2	332	379	3	4
Subtotal	865	768	155	281	16	13	12	5	2,788	3,103	8	16	2,473	3,186	85	72
Other																
Tenured	0	1	0	0	0	0	0	0	3	4	0	0	1	0	0	0
On Track	1	3	0	1	0	0	0	0	16	28	0	0	12	30	0	0
Not on Track	140	99	25	23	3	1	1	0	470	505	8	3	475	537	25	17
Not Available	10	9	1	1	0	0	0	0	28	30	0	0	37	27	0	0
Missing	55	39	3	2	0	0	1	0	85	59	2	0	165	185	3	2
Subtotal	206	151	29	27	3	1	2	0	602	626	10	3	690	779	28	19

AAMC Faculty Roster
December 31, 2011

Note: This table excludes 127 faculty with missing sex data.

6

Table 4. Women in Medical School Administrative Positions

	1975-76		1991-92		2009	
	Total	*Women*	*Total*	*Women*	*Total*	*Women*
Deans	119	0	126	5*	1171	13
Senior Associate Deans	N/A	N/A	N/A	10	402	113
Associate Deans	382	13(3.4%)	772	114 (14.7%)	1024	365 (36%)
Assistant Deans	249	29 (11.7%)	405	102 (25.1%)	603	285 (47%)

Source: Directory of American Medical Education, 1991-92. Washington, D.C.: Association of American Medical Colleges.
Source: Women in Academic Medicine Statistics. Washington, D.C.: Association of American Medical Colleges, 1993.

*As of November 1993 (includes two interim deans).

(chief human resources officer) rather than CEO (chief executive officer), COO (chief operating officer), CFO (chief financial officer) or CMO (chief medical officer).

This gender inequality issue is compounded by the fact that few physicians of either gender are tapped for senior hospital management roles. According to a 2009 paper published by Gunderman and Kantor[12], only 235 (fewer than 4 percent) of 6500 hospitals in the US at the time were headed by physicians of either gender.

Insurance Companies

The situation is no better in insurance companies. Of the five top health insurance companies (Aetna, Cigna, Humana, United Healthcare, and Wellpoint), none are currently headed by physicians (Dr. William McGuire was the former head of United Healthcare).

Pharmaceutical and Biotech Companies

There is no published data regarding leadership roles for women physicians in the pharmaceutical or biotechnology industries. However, a 2007 landmark Healthcare Business Association (HBA) E.D.G.E. paper titled "The Progress of Women Executives in Pharmaceuticals and Biotechnology: A Leadership Benchmarking Study" did track the career progress of women in general[13]. The research was sponsored by Booz Allen Hamilton,Novartis, Sanofi-aventis, Wyeth, Abbott Laboratories, AstraZeneca, Celgene, Ernst & Young, Johnson & Johnson and Merck & Co and used insights from three study arms: 82 senior executives who gave in-depth interviews, 237 mid-level managers who responded to a comprehensive Internet survey, and human resources data and questionnaires submitted by 12 of the top 50 life sciences companies.

Based on findings from E.D.G.E participants, women hold 17 percent of senior management positions in the life sciences industry. This number varies widely among firms, topping out at 57 percent; several companies had no women in senior management at all. In middle management, female representation is higher, with women occupying roughly one-third of positions. This number is consistent between biotechnology and pharmaceutical companies and across companies in Europe and the United States. Within all life sciences companies, the greatest representation of women middle managers is in research and development (37 percent) and corporate functions (34 percent). The lowest representation is in information technology, where women hold only 12 percent of middle management positions.

Why a glass ceiling for physicians of both genders?

Several phenomena seem to account for the glass ceiling experienced by both male and female physicians. First, there is the poor public relations image that physicians have had in terms of their business acumen. Many physicians themselves feel they are bad at business; they have the perception that they cannot handle the financial management of a large organization and could never aspire to COO or CEO roles.

Second is the pervasive concern by non-physicians that doctors who have the power to influence patient decision-making will place their own financial self-interests ahead of the well-being of their patients and steer them toward expensive procedures that do not necessarily create better outcomes[12].

A third reason for so few physician managers at the top is based on a historical perspective. Earlier in this century there were far more physician CEOs in hospitals; in 1935, physicians were in charge of 35 percent of all hospitals[14]. However, World War II brought a transition point as a number of non-physicians entered the medical administration corps. At war's end, many of these men trained in running hospitals during the war were eager to do the same in the civilian world. At the same time, the technology of health care had increased and most physicians were willing to relinquish their administrator roles, preferring to devote their time to the scientific and clinical side of medicine.

For years, physicians who remained in hospital administration tended to be retired military men, doctors who had encountered physical problems, and even some who couldn't succeed in private practice. When they became administrators, they were often shunted off into clinically focused areas such as education, medical staff credentialing and hiring, and quality assurance issues.

In 1970, a Fortune magazine cover story[16] warned the country that "much of US medical care, particularly the everyday business of preventing and treating routine illness is inferior in quality, wastefully dispensed and inequitably financed." That same year a Fortune editorial declared: "the time has come for radical change...the management of medical care is too important to leave to doctors who are, after all, not managers to begin with."

Nineteen eighty-two marked the beginning of Paul Starr's "social transformation of American medicine". In the final chapter of his Pulitzer Prize winning book with the same title[17], he expressed concerns about the coming of the corporation and the re-focus from the 1970's emphasis on "health care planning" to "health care marketing" just one decade later. He was obviously prescient.

Indeed health care in the US since then has become increasingly perceived in terms of an economic service, organized and delivered through large, complex managed systems.

This new paradigm altered traditional positions of power and influence within health care as the power of large corporate providers and large purchasers grew, and the dominance of physicians and professional organizations diminished. Very quickly, non-physician business school graduates began displacing graduates of public health schools as well as doctors in top echelons of medical care organizations, taking on mainstream management roles, including financial, strategic planning, and policy making responsibilities. This same trend (i.e., physicians as traditional medical directors, non-physicians as operational managers) was seen not only in hospitals, but also in most insurance companies and managed care organizations.

Despite the fact that there has been lots of discussion about including physician leaders in more senior positions in all aspects of health care, those at the highest levels are still predominantly non-physicians and mostly male.

Regardless of how reform ultimately evolves, the 2010 passage of the Affordable Care Act has set in motion disruption of the status quo that presents both challenges and opportunities for physicians interested in leveraging their expertise to influence health care delivery as medical managers. More than ever, a career in medical management is a positive choice for female as well as male physicians.

In addition to having excellent physicians at the core of the health care system clinically, there is a compelling case for a physician-executive who possesses the skills and knowledge about the organization of medical care and can act as liaison among all those with an interest in medicine, including patients, health care providers, insurers, economists, and other administrators.

In a 2011 paper, Amanda Goodall[18] found that the highest rated hospitals according to the US News and World Report's "Best Hospitals" ranking were led disproportionately by physicians. Goodall acknowledged that because there is no other hard evidence published about the relative merits of having physicians and non-physician managers in leadership positions, her discussion merely starts the empirical process. As Tracy Duberman, PhD wrote in a recent PEJ Journal[19], physician leaders in 2012 and beyond will be measured by "the results they achieve, the value or efficiency with which they achieve good outcomes, and improvements in performance resulting from a focus on teamwork through superior coordination, information sharing, and teaming across disciplines."

With the health care delivery system evolving faster than ever, today's physician leaders not only need to have a broad base of skills and knowledge (e.g. understanding the current requirements for physician reporting, health care financing, accountable care organizations, clinical process improvement, utilization management, clinical decision support systems, team based care and more), but must also be strategic thinkers and effective communicators.

What Makes a Good Manager?

Generally speaking, physicians and managers have different perspectives, goals, and objectives. Physicians are trained to focus on individual patients, their needs and problems. Physicians' decision-making tends to be methodical and highly rationalized, often requiring a great deal of autonomy. On the other hand, health care managers are trained to focus on the organization and its problems as well as on larger socioeconomic issues of the environment. While the decision-making of managers is careful and ideally rational, it generally requires collaboration, often without having all the information they would like and nearly always with budget issues in mind. Clearly, many of the skills required to be a good clinician (such as the ability to weigh factors involved in a decision, to put into perspective the relationship between cost and the impact of a decision on a patient's health, and to recognize when health care services can do no more for a patient) are transferable to the role of manager.

However, some skills must be newly learned for the role of manager. As the professional leader, the manager becomes the activator of the organization's central nervous system. He or she must diagnose the organization as an environment and act in it as a leadership figure to whom and about whom subordinates have significant feelings. The leader must motivate, meaning he or she must get things done through others, while simultaneously maintaining a balance among conflicting interests in the organization. He or she must manage change in an orderly fashion.

In practice, a difficult patient can be referred. Management generally does not have the same luxury. Problems keep coming no matter how many you already have. Rarely can you refer a difficult issue to someone else. While delegation can help and in fact is a necessary skill for the manager, it does not relieve him or her of responsibility. Most important, in management one does not get daily strokes from patients. One must derive satisfaction from the knowledge that a particular decision or program has changed the care patients receive in some positive way.

Management Credentials: An Ongoing Controversy

As health care organizations are forced to balance complex quality and cost issues, talented physician executives are in increasing demand. Although there is general agreement that physician executives should have strong clinical credentials, a continuing question and controversy in medical management is the nature of the educational background that is best for a successful management career. Certainly the traditional hospital/clinic arrangement, with total separation of administrative and clinical matters, is rapidly becoming obsolete. The issue is particularly sensitive for physicians who have already spent a number of years in medical practice or even medical management. Will informal training suffice, or are physician executives faced with the necessity of obtaining formal degrees in management?

Some large physician groups like the Cleveland and Mayo Clinics have explicitly introduced leadership training for their doctors, generally affiliating with local business schools[20]. Likewise, management and leadership education has been incorporated into some medical degree programs[21-23]. At the time of the original 1995 publication of "Women in Medicine and Management", there were few physicians with MBAs. As recently as the late 1990's there were only 5 or 6 joint MD/MBA programs in the US. By 2011, there were 65. Statistics about these joint programs are limited, but Dr. Maria Y. Chandler, a pediatrician with an MBA who is associate professor in the medical and business school at the University of California at Irvine and president of the Association of MD/MBA Programs, estimates as many as 500 students are currently enrolled in these combined programs[24].

Despite these trends, we will probably continue to have two separate groups of physicians in management: those who are less interested in formal degrees and those who see their careers in a longitudinal sense and who will want to go back to the university setting to get a "ticket" to go with their MDs.

Whether one goes the university route or learns only on the job, management, like medicine, is ever-changing, and skills and knowledge will need to be constantly supplemented by extensive reading of the pertinent management literature and attendance at appropriate seminars and courses. A new literature has emerged, focusing on key competencies required to be an effective physician leader[25-26].

Do Women Make Better Managers than Men Do?

In the almost two decades since the publication of the first version of this monograph, women have made incredible strides in terms of the level of formal education achieved and numbers within the workforce. Yet relatively few have risen to the highest levels in politics, Fortune 500 companies or health care organizations—public or private.

The commonly cited reason, apart from sexism, for their poor showing in leadership positions has been that women choose not to be leaders, that they lack interest and skill in leadership, and that they choose to devote their time to their families rather than concentrating their attention on professional advancement. While past studies justifying male physicians as administrators declared that men like wielding power more than women do, there is more agreement today that when women have an opportunity to be decision makers as medical managers, they enjoy the role[27]. A 2011 survey conducted by McKinsey [28] showed that women's interest in being leaders increases as they move from entry level positions to middle management.

Not only do women enjoy management roles, they make excellent leaders. In fact, in a 2008 PEW survey[29], the public rated women better than or equal to men in 7 of 8 leadership traits. Dr. Alice Eagly, one of the top scholars on gender and leadership agrees. Her studies show that women are more likely than men to possess the leadership qualities associated with success. According to Eagly, women are more transformational than men—they care more about developing their followers, they listen to them and stimulate them to think "outside the box," they are more inspirational, and they are more ethical[30].

When David Ross, assistant professor of management at Columbia's Business School and Cristian Dezso, his colleague at the University of Maryland, studied the top 1,500 U.S. companies over 15 years ending in 2006, they found that the firms with women at the top performed significantly better. This was especially true for the firms that put high emphasis on innovation. Such firms often belong to creative industries and tend to spend disproportionately on research and development.[31] The study provides evidence for the existence of the so-called "female management style", which holds that female executives tend to manage in a more democratic way, as opposed to the more autocratic approach associated with the stereotypical male boss. That democratic style fosters creativity, teamwork and desire to solve problems.

Dr. Bernard Bass, who developed the current theory of transformational leadership, predicts that in the future women leaders will dominate simply because they are better suited to 21st century leadership/management than are men.[32]

2012 and Beyond

In spite of Bass' hopeful prediction, and evidence supporting the quality or even superiority of women as managers, men continue to dominate leadership positions. The question is: what is preventing highly qualified women from reaching the top? According to Dr. Eagly and others, women have to overcome obstacles to attain leadership positions, while men are offered a "free pass." Eagly claims that as a society, our image of a leader is "male," and so we more often select or promote men. Men still tend to control the hiring and favor men over women. We are simply reluctant to change the status quo. Unfortunately, when pollsters ask, "Is the United States ready for a woman President?" the majority still answer "No".

This monograph sets out to document the career paths that some successful women physician managers have taken. Ten (Drs. Cary, Hammond, Calmes, Batchlor, Petersen, LeTourneu, Yaremchuk, Ford, Gabow and Shlian) were contributors to the original 1995 publication. In this update they continue to share their experiences over the past 17 years. Fourteen (Drs. Pescovitz, Parker, Young, Komives, Roldan, Haseltine, Maglioto, Sennholz, Ferguson, Terrell, Asmar, McCormick, Strahlman, and Goonan) are new contributors. All these women have found success in many different areas of medical management. They include corporate medical directors, managed care executives, managers within government, the pharmaceutical industry, academic leaders, hospital executives, and entrepreneurs.

All of these women say they enjoy management, that they opted for their management positions as "part of their overall career enhancement." Most say that their desire to be managers grew out of a desire to be policy makers, to have a chance to provide top management support for medical practitioners, and to influence the larger picture (how groups of patients receive care and also the environment in which services are delivered). In 1995 only one woman noted the emerging importance of professional roles in managing the technical complexity of cost containment. Today everyone agrees that this is a priority.

Whatever the reasons for having chosen to transition from clinical medicine to medical management, all the stories here are compelling. Readers (both female and male) embarking on a management career, or even those already on a career path, may learn from the failures as well as the successes that each of the contributors to this monograph has found along the way.

REFERENCES

1. Women Physicians Congress, August 2011 A Profile & History of Women in Medicine, AMA

2. Bennett, Leslie "Women and the Leadership Gap" Newsweek Magazine, March 5, 2012

3. Women in National Parliaments- data compiled by the Inter-Parliamentary Union, December, 2011 accessed at: http://www.ipu.org/wmn-e/classif.htm

4. Brown AJ, Swinyard W. Ogle J. Women in academic medicine: A report of focus groups and questionnaires with conjoint analysis J Womens Health (Larchmt. 2003; 12:999-1008

5. Leonard JC, Ellsbury KE, Gender and interest in academic careers by first and third year residents Acad Med 1996;71:502-504

6. Leadley J. Women in US Academic Medicine Statistics and Benchmarking Report 2008-2009 accessed: http://www.aamc.org/members/gwims/statistics/stats09/wimstatisticsreport2009.pdf -Accessed September 21, 2010

7. Ash, AS, Carr PL, Goldstein R., Friedman, RH Compensation and Advancement of women in academic medicine: Is there equity? Ann Int Med 2004;141:205-212

8. Nonnemaker L. Women physicians in academic medicine: New insights from cohort studies N Eng J Med 2000;342: 399-405

9. Reed, Darcy A, MD, MPH; Felicity Enders PhD, Rachel Lindoe, Martha McClees and Keith D Lindor, MD Gender Differences in Academic Productivity and Leadership Appointments of Physicians Throughout Academic Careers Academic Medicine Vol 86, No 1, January 2011

10. Borges, Nicole J. PhD; Navarro, Anita MED; Grover, Amelia C, MD: Women Physicians: Choosing a Career in Academic Medicine Academic Medicine: January 2012- Vol 87, Issue 1 pp 105-114 doi

11. Branin, Joan Julia, Director Center for Health and Aging, Chair Masters in Health Administration, University of LaVerne "Career Attainment Among Healthcare Executives-Is the Gender Gap Narrowing?" 2009 Forum on Public Policy

12. Gunderman, Richard, MD, PhD and Kantor, Steven L. MD Perspectives: Educating Physicians to Lead Hospitals, Academic Medicine, October 2009, Vol 84, Issue 10 pp1348-1351

13. 2007 Healthcare Business Association (HBA. E.D.G.E. paper: "The Progress of Women Executives in Pharmaceuticals and Biotechnology: A Leadership Benchmarking Study

14. Maher, Maggie, Healthcare fellow at The Century Foundation: Money Driven Medicine: The real reason healthcare costs so much, Collins, May 2006

15. MacEachern MT "Hospital Organization and Management" Chicago, Ill Physicians Record Co, 1935

16. "Our Ailing Medical System: It's Time to Operate". Fortune Magazine (New York, Harper & Row). January 1970

17. Starr, Paul The Social Transformation of American Medicine.: the rise of a sovereign profession and the making of a vast industry, Basic Books, June, 1984

18. Goodall, Amanda Physician Leaders and Hospital Performance Discussion Paper # 5830 ISA and Cass Business School, July 21, 2011

19. Duberman, Tracy PhD Developing Physician Leaders Today Using the 70/20/10 Rule PEJ September- October 2011 pp66-68

20. Stoller, J.K., Berkowitz, E., and Bailin, P.L. (2007. Physician management and leadership education at the Cleveland Clinic Foundation: program impact and experience over 14 years. Journal of Medical Practice Management, 22:237-42.

21. Fairchild, DG, Benjamin, EM, Gifford DR, and Hout, SJ (2004. Physician leadership: Enhancing the career development of academic physician administrators and leaders Academic Medicine 79; 214-218

22. Stern, D.T. and Papadakis, M (2006. The developing physician- becoming a professional New England Journal of Medicine, 355: 1794-1799.

23. Baker, CJ and Hafferty, FW 2007 Professionalism New Eng J 356:966

24. Freudebhem, Milton "Adjusting, More MDs Add MBAs" NY Times, Sept 5, 2011

25. Chaudry, J., Jain A., McKenzie S. and Scwartz, RW (2008. Physician leadership: the competency of change. Journal of Surgical Education, 65: 213-220

26. Stoller, J.K. (2008 Developing physician-leaders: A Call to action Journal of General Internal Medicine, 24: 876-878

27. MacEachern MT Hospital Organization and Management Chicago, Ill Physicians Record Co, 1935

28. Barsh, Joanna and Yee, Lareina "Changing Companie's Minds About Women" Mckinsey 2011 survey. Accessed at: http://www.mckinsey.com/careers/women/~/media/Reports/Women/Changing_companies_minds_about_women.ashx

29. PEW Research Center Publications, August 25, 2008, Accessed at: http://pewresearch.org/pubs/932/men-or-women-whos-the-better-leader

30. Alice H. Eagley and Carli, Linda L. Through the Labyrinth: The Truth About How Women Become Leaders (Center for Public Leadership. Harvard Business School Press (October 16, 2007)

31. When women rank high, companies profit" HR Magazine, August 2009

32. Bass, Bernard M. and Riggio, Ronald E. Transformational Leadership (2nd ed), Psychological Press Taylor & Francis Group, 2006.

GOVERNMENT

CHAPTER TWO

Sex and Science Drove My Life

by Florence Haseltine, MD, PhD

For me, a lifetime of accomplishment began decades ago with the simplest of scientific questions: why? The solution lay in the two driving forces of my life— Sex and Science.

A child blessed with deep curiosity about the origin of gender, I didn't expect easy answers. I wanted the entire scientific story, and determined then and there to unscramble the toughest mysteries myself.

As a biophysicist, obstetrician-gynecologist, reproductive endocrinologist, National Institutes of Health research head, professional journal editor, best-selling novelist, inventor, and advocate for women's health, I guess you could say that I have cut a wide swath through science, medicine and government since my early years as an inquisitive youngster living on a scientific outpost.

My efforts to include women in clinical trials have forever changed medicine. Along the way, I have also penned a best-selling book, earned several patents, created award-winning computer applications, set up my own business, and raised two daughters who are already making significant contributions to their fields.

And it all began with an inquisitive moment in a desert town.

The beginnings

In China Lake, California, a remote military outpost where my father was among the many research scientists, I was an intensely curious youngster, desperate to understand the mysteries that surrounded me. I peppered my physicist father with endless questions, demanding to know why there had to be both boys and girls. Even though he was an uncommunicative man, he made a few attempts but then exasperated, answered with his own question. "When you grow up, why don't you figure it out?" The challenge set me on a lifelong quest that was unrelenting – and often difficult.

Struggling to come to terms with my inability to read, which I now attribute to dyslexia unknown at the time, as a youngster I gravitated to math and science. By the age of 12, I had decided that I would one day become a doctor. But first, I had to contend with the unremitting boredom of a closeted community that was removed by distance and geography from the rest of the world. A literal oasis in the middle of California's Mojave Desert, China Lake was rich in scientists, researchers, and natural beauty but impoverished in things to do. I harnessed my own brainpower for entertainment, and vowed to leave the desert behind as soon as possible.

Within a few days of my high school graduation, I took Greeley's words literally and boarded a bus headed West for the University of California at Davis. My summer studies in basic biology, conducted by the National Science Foundation, opened an entirely new world of scientific possibilities; a chance to begin addressing the queries that dogged me.

Education

From Davis, I went to the University of California at Berkeley, where I was the rare female majoring in biophysics. Studying among skeptical male classmates, I proved my doubters wrong for the first of many times. Not only did I earn my degree, but I moved across the country to continue my studies at the ultimate bastion of male scientific achievement, the Massachusetts Institute of Technology. There, I earned a PhD in biophysics in 1970 and married a classmate. When I learned I'd have to remain at MIT while my husband finished his work on his PhD, I got a divorce and moved to New York, determined to deliver on my childhood pledge to become a physician. I studied at the Albert Einstein College of Medicine, happy to find accepting peers bound by a passion for "the art of medicine".

Several years later, I interned at the University of Pennsylvania, completed my residency at Boston Hospital for Women (Brigham and Women's Hospital), and was board certified in obstetrics and gynecology as well as in reproductive endocrinology. I became an assistant and associate professor in the

Department of Ob/Gyn and Pediatrics at Yale University.

During my time in Boston I met a fellow scientist-physics professor Alan Chodos- who would become my second husband. With time and infertility treatments, we had two daughters. Anna, the oldest is a Gerontologist at UCSF and Elizabeth is an Associate Director of the OxBow, an artist residency program. During a sabbatical year at Yale, I decided that I lacked a proper understanding of business, a problem I remedied by studying strategic planning and business development at the Yale School of Organization and Management.

At Yale, I served on several academic committees, often as the sole woman member, distinguishing myself as a tireless, if outspoken, advocate for women's advancement and professional development. I also set down my experiences as a physician in a novel that went on to be a top seller. In "Woman Doctor", I fictionalized the very real personal and professional challenges I had faced while becoming an MD.

Finally able to devote my full attention to the study of sex differences, I won research grants from the Center at the National Institutes of Health , the same Center I would later lead. I focused on in vitro fertilization and later broadened my scope to explore the behavioral impact fertility treatments had on couples.

Revolutionizing research

I quickly unearthed a serious oversight in the manner data for medical investigations was collected. Because clinical trials and biomedical research routinely included only male subjects, the ways women responded to illness and disease were virtually unknown. Deeply concerned about the implications for female patients, I vowed to change the system. Happily, my efforts have forever altered medical research.

In 1985, I was tapped to become the Director of the Center for Population Research at the National Institutes of Child Health and Human Development at the National Institutes of Health. The commute from my New Haven home to my new Washington, DC office created a personal challenge, but it was worth it. In my role, I successfully influenced the direction of national reproductive health policy. During my tenure, the office's budget rose to more than $350 million annually, funding a wide variety of projects—clinical trials for novel contraceptives for men and women, research on early pregnancy and implantation mechanisms, support for under-appreciated yet critical health challenges facing women including pelvic organ prolapse, studies of population dynamics and impacts on health as well as the relationship between maternal literacy and children's academic achievements in resource poor settings.

In 1990, I established the Society for Women's Health Research (SWHR), becoming its first president. The organization soon documented the clear sexual bias plaguing biomedical research. SWHR's findings prompted a Government Accounting Office (GAO) investigation into research methodology, highlighting the failure of most studies to comply with National Institutes of Health guidelines mandating diverse clinical trial populations. Determining that most such studies violated these NIH requirements, the government established new policies that set inviolable new rules for broad-based data. To coordinate the research and monitor compliance, NIH created the Office of Research on Women's Health (ORWH).

Throughout, I worked to expand my message beyond the research community. As editor-in-chief of the Journal of Women's Health, I reported on the state of scientific inquiry. I also edited the comprehensive report Women's Health Research: A Medical and Policy Primer published by the Society for Women's Health Research and led its follow-up studies. Additionally, I served as a founding member of the Organization for the Study of Sex Differences (OSSD), an international society that coordinates connections between basic and clinical scientists from multiple scientific disciplines with shared interests in sex difference-related topics.

My interest in the area of mentoring is not simply limited to the fact that one should be mentored. I am very interested in the many different ways people mentor as well as why people are willing to be mentors. My articles[1,2,3] span four decades, from 1977 to 2005. Again, these articles demonstrate my keen interest in the advancement of young people.

I have been fortunate to have been honored for my contributions to reproductive medicine and women's health. A frequent speaker, I have won awards from professional societies, advocacy groups, and the federal government for my public service, and I was elected to the Institute of Medicine. I am proud of the fact that I have been credited for the GAO's success in building data on women and minorities into its clinical research, which was re-assessed favorably in 2000 and for the loan repayment program now funded by many NIH institutes which helps medical researchers pay off their debt.

Current Projects

Now Emerita Director at the Center for Population Research at the Eunice

Kennedy Shriver National Institute for Child Health and Human Development (NICHD) of the National Institutes of Health (NIH), I continue to break new ground.

I helped architect the RAISE Project (Recognizing the Achievements of Women in Science, Medicine and Engineering), devoted to enhancing the status of professional women in science, technology, engineering, mathematics and medicine. RAISE provides valuable information and analysis of national and international scientific awards and award recipients disaggregated by sex. RAISE is being considered as a Department of State "best practice" program to help inform other nations as part of a global agenda on advancement of women in science.

Ever curious, I tested entrepreneurship with the launch of Haseltine Systems Corporation in 1995 to design products for people with disabilities. I earned two patents for my Haseltine Flyer, a container that protects wheel chairs during air travel.

Two more patents on an internet application, granted in 2007, provides shoppers with a customized system that allows them to see and share photos of prospective clothing purchases with others. I recently released a smart phone application, Embryo, which allows users to manipulate 3D images and videos of human eggs, sperm and fertilization from the famous Carnegie Embryo Collection. I facilitated the collaboration among the National Library of Medicine, the National Museum of Health and Medicine, and NICHD that spawned application. Especially fun was that I not only conceptualized Embryo, but also acquired the programming skills needed to build it, ultimately earning a 2011 National Library of Medicine honor.

My curiosity has taken me a long way from a desert town that has since all but vanished, but it has returned me – time and again – to the wonder of science. Questions, I insist, can still change the world. I still want to know why are there two sexes.

REFERENCES

1. Haseltine FP: Why be a role model when you can be a mentor? Women's Leadership and Authority in the Health Professions at Santa Cruz, 1977.

2. Shapiro EC, Haseltine FP, Rowe MP: Moving up: role models, mentors, and the "patron system." Sloan Management Rev 1978; 19:51-58.

3. Haseltine FP: Why Be A Mentor? In: DC Fort (ed). A Hand Up - Women Mentoring Women In Science. Washington, DC: Association for Women In Science (AWIS) Publisher, 2005; pp.353-366.

CHAPTER THREE

Boundroid

by Margaret (Maggi) Cary, MD, MBA, MPH

Boundroid[SM] is not a word you will find in any standard dictionary. If you could, its definition would read Boundroid *(n): A person who works at the interface among people, groups and/or cultures to intentionally create change; a particular form of change agent.* Boundroids possess innate and acquired abilities to effect change. They cross personal, social and organizational barriers that separate individuals or groups of people, preventing the free exchange of energy, ideas and opportunities. Boundroids are ubiquitous, but difficult to recognize if you are blind to their skills and unable to pick up their distinctive trail.

Over sixteen years have passed since the first edition of Women in Medicine and Management: A Mentoring Guide. More women are in medicine, dentistry and veterinary medicine. Some graduating classes have more women than men.

As I wrote in the first edition, I wanted to be a physician since fourth grade. I loved science and wanted to help people. I took some side roads and eventually left direct patient care for management. I preferred working in groups rather than alone. I have been fortunate in being a lifelong learner, enjoying "knowledge transfer" with others and in having many, many people who believed in me and helped me. After completing medical school and the Santa Rosa, California residency in Family Medicine, I managed my own private practice and then co-directed an emergency department in a ski resort. Some of my other activities include turning around a money-losing occupational medicine clinic, earning a master's in business administration (MBA) and developing and co-anchoring a nationally aired Public Broadcasting System coproduction, "The Health Care Puzzle." At the time of the publication of the previous edition of this book, I was a member of President Clinton's Administration, as one of Secretary Shalala's Regional Directors in Health and Human Services. I intended to stay one term. The job was one of the most challenging and rewarding jobs I had ever had, so I stayed for the second term. As the second term was winding down, I started looking for another job.

In 2000, the president of Acueity, a medical device start-up in the Bay Area, and

I began discussing my joining the company. I had co-authored a seminal text on telehealth, *Telemedicine and Telehealth: Principles, Policies, Performance and Pitfalls* (which continues to sell), and the president wanted me to bring my knowledge of medical technology, medicine, public policy and communications skills to Acueity. I would stay in Denver and commute to San Francisco when I wasn't visiting clients. I had lived in the Bay Area for some of my high school and college years and returned to Sonoma County for my residency training.

I thought this new commute would be an opportunity to reconnect with my family and friends. Moreover, the product intrigued me. Acueity sold micro endoscopes with a diameter of less than a millimeter. The market edge was the patented optics, created by two cinematographers that provided detailed resolution of the smallest details. The initial use was for ductoscopy to diagnose ductal carcinoma *in situ*. I thought of additional uses. I could use my skills and contacts to further the company's goals. The optimal job for a Boundroid – the intersection of medicine, Federal government, business and public policy.

Find a need and fill it, whatever it takes.

In late 2000, the tech bubble imploded and funding dried up. One of the partners in the healthcare communications company we had hired asked me to join as medical director, continuing to live in Denver, but now commuting to Philadelphia. Living in Denver and working in the Bay Area had not been as easy as I'd thought it would be. I was tired of being on the road. Connecting with my friends was difficult, given weekday traffic and the distances. The few family members in the Bay Area were nearly 100 miles away. Most evenings I returned to an empty hotel room, eating fast food.

Why, then, would I even *consider* a job with a longer commute between Denver and Philadelphia—a place where I knew no one and wasn't familiar with the culture? Because here was another opportunity to be a Boundroid. The new position would combine my expertise as clinician, Federal government employee, writer, policy analyst and public speaker. I could learn the details of marketing, advertising and public relations, all of which measure their effectiveness with research, much as medicine does.

I enjoyed the people I worked with – the creativity and camaraderie – but had a hard time, in the end, promoting another "me too" drug when we had over 40 million uninsured people in the United States. The friendliness of the staff, and the extensive wine by the glass selection of the Penn's View Inn, where I stayed, did not compensate for eating dinner alone and returning to another empty hotel room. I wanted to sleep in my own bed. So when Donna Marshall, president of the Colorado Business Group on Health, began recruiting me as her chief medical officer, I listened. I liked Donna (and still do) and wanted to return to mission-driven work, where I fully believed in what I was doing. I decided to return to Colorado.

In 2003, I received an offer from the Veterans Health Administration (VHA) in Washington, DC to develop and implement VA+Choice, a complicated program to allow Medicare-eligible Veterans to use their Medicare benefits at VA facilities, purportedly developed on the back of a napkin by the (then) Secretaries of Health and Human Services and the Department of Veterans Affairs with their respective Under Secretaries. I had enjoyed working at Health and Human Services; the Federal government's mission resonated with me and I enjoyed working with my colleagues. The VHA post required a physician with a background in health policy, public health, and business, who also had excellent communication skills – a small universe in 2003. This was another chance to build on the skills I had developed in my previous jobs.

I was committed to Denver and my 20-year history living there, to my family in Boulder, swearing I would only leave my house feet first in a box. The VHA post meant moving to Washington, DC. I looked at strengths and weaknesses, opportunities and threats, for each choice and ultimately decided to move. The chance to be a Boundroid again was irresistible.

I hit the ground running, learning about VA's electronic health record (EHR), information technology (IT) system, coding and billing. I enjoy being on a vertical learning curve. Bob Perreault, the man who hired me, was an excellent boss. He gave me free rein to meet with whomever I wished at VA without going up through the chain of command. At the time I didn't realize how uncommon this is in bureaucracies. Bob introduced me to VA's leaders who could help. He was one of the best bosses I have ever had. We trusted each other, an essential piece of an effective and productive relationship.

As part of accountability I was evaluated by an external organizational development consultant, who wrote:

> "Maggi has done a phenomenal job of laying out the implementation strategy and the elements for the program. Most folks focus only on the process pieces of the program, i.e., how the system is to work, and they normally minimize or ignore the vision building, the involvement of stakeholders and partners, the development of staff and the marketing and PR work that will help guarantee success. Maggi has taken all of that into account. I think you will find her efforts very impressive."

My previous experiences and expertise meshed well in this post. I came in early and stayed late, working on weekends.

After the Health Insurance Portability and Accountability Act of 1996 (HIPAA) was enacted I renamed VA+Choice to VAAdvantage, the first Medicare+Choice program. Then, for reasons relating to leadership changes at the top in 2004 (one of the risks in Federal government positions), VAAdvantage was shelved.

In 2006, I moved from the business to the clinical side of the Veterans Health Administration to manage over 20 Field Advisory Committees of medical specialties. The Committees had languished for years. My job was to engage them with the Office of Specialty Care Services, their home office. I asked Committee members what they would like from the Washington, DC policy office. One item was management and leadership training.

Drawing on my private sector experience, I created and delivered one- to two-day physician leadership development workshops around the country, all with outstanding evaluations. VHA's standard evaluation takes six weeks and I wanted a quicker turnaround, so I developed my own assessment, collated the responses and then shared with all who wanted it. I enjoyed the work and wanted to include other faculty.

Find a need and fill it, whatever it takes.

In 2004, while I was at VHA, my youngest brother was driving supply trucks for the US military in Iraq, the same trucks targeted for Improvised Explosive Devices, or IEDs. During his first month, his eleven-year-old daughter found her mother, Kelly, comatose. The daughter awakened her sixteen-year-old sister and called 911. Kelly had experienced a brain bleed and lingered for a couple of weeks. During most of her hospital stay her open brain was swathed in bandages, following the craniotomy to decrease her intracranial pressure (the pressure inside her skull). She never awakened. After she died, my other brothers, my stepmother and her husband and I stepped in to care for my nieces while their father completed his contract.

I was now one of a group responsible for the health and well-being of two young girls while their father had a risky job far away. My summer's month with them was one of the high points in my life. We made pies from the apples in our yard, saw films and held a birthday party for my younger niece's twelfth. I thought about their needs over my own. I remember having something – I don't remember what it was – that one of them wanted. Without thinking I gave it to her. I did not weigh the pros and cons. I just handed it to her.

Find a need and fill it, whatever it takes.

The repeated theme in my career has been to find a need and fill it, whatever it takes, often a unique need or a unique way to fill it. My first Boundroid experience was in 1983 when I turned around a Denver clinic. I had moved from California to Colorado. I needed a job and chose the one that was most appealing to me. Rose Hospital was in the vanguard of buying medical practices. My preference was the clinic in downtown Denver in a new building with designer furniture, but another physician was hired for that position. I was stuck with the occupational and general medicine clinic in a run-down house in industrial Denver. Depending upon which way the wind blew, I smelled cat food, lamb or fertilizer.

Rather than just accepting the situation, I began thinking larger, thinking tactically and strategically. Industrial injuries were our cash cow. Local drop-ins were not as profitable. Caring for them was good for community support and I enjoyed my patients. Without knowing exactly what I was doing at the time, I visited the foremen at the factories who referred those hurt on the job for medical care. I gave classes at the factories on preventing back injuries and industrial safety. This led to more business. I created occupational and physician therapy offices in the clinic basement so that our patients spent less time off work to have their therapies. They did not have to travel to the main hospital located several miles south and on the other side of the freeway. The hospital still captured the revenue.

Find a need and fill it, whatever it takes.

Keep in mind that filling these needs may have unexpected consequences, positive and negative. In the 1980's turning around an occupational medicine clinic offered a wide open future, and my work was in the industrial part of Denver, a perfect location. After transforming a clinic that was in the red for three years into a profit-winning operation within ninety days, I negotiated a contract with a lower base, but with bonuses based on billed charges, not collected charges. My yearly salary rose. I was transferred to another location in a working-class residential Denver area, with lots of close-by private doctor offices as competition. Unfortunately, I couldn't build another successful medical clinic here. Most of the neighborhood residents worked during the day and went to clinics closer to their jobs or to free clinics. The hospital was reluctant to open on weekends or evenings and, truthfully, so was I. Management changed at the hospital and the new manager had different ideas that I wasn't sure would work in the environment. I finally left and the clinic closed.

Because of my turn-around success with the occupational medicine clinic, the chief executive officers (CEOs) of Denver's competing clinics pursued me to join their businesses. I chose the more financially successful, thinking I would again have both management and patient care roles. Instead, I was put into a line job, which meant I was simply another physician seeing patients and completing the appropriate on-the-job injury forms. I had no input into building the business or in client outreach. Worse yet, I had to punch in and out on a timecard and was paid an hourly rate. This was not the job I signed up for. I completed my contract and resigned.

I wanted to reinvent myself and so I returned to university to earn an MBA. I founded a consulting company. I read about the Miles Institute for Physician Patient Communication (now the Institute for Healthcare Communication) in the Wall Street Journal, and joined the first train-the-trainer course, delivering workshops in Colorado.

Today, as mentioned above, I develop, manage and teach at physician leadership development workshops for VA physicians. I am a credentialed executive coach. I developed and teach the Personal Essay/Narrative Medicine course at Georgetown University School of Medicine. I deliver a yearly leadership development workshop at George Washington University School of Medicine. I am a Professional Member of the National Speakers Association and speak about physician leadership development as well as about using the coaching approach in management and leadership.

Find a need and fill it, whatever it takes.

One key to success at any job is to listen to the folks who are already there. Ask what they like, what could be improved and what they'd like to see happen. Relationships are the foundation for all we do. Life is a balancing act—the balance of risk and security. As a lifelong learner, I look for new ideas, for new ways of being and doing. I'm fortunate to have a life where one experience leads to the next.

My three requirements for employment are

- Do meaningful work,
- Make enough to live on, and
- Work with constructive, positive people.

In the first edition of Women in Medicine and Management I offered the following, which still hold.

- Have a goal in life.

- Be authentic.

- Speak the truth.

- Join a community.

- Make friends and acquaintances and maintain the relationships you develop. Be interested in the person, not the position.

- Listen, listen, listen – especially important in a new job. Develop exemplary listening skills.

- Figure out who your boss is and what your boss wants, and do it. Do a quality job on time.

- Let folks (especially your boss) know what you're doing while maintaining humility.

- Share power.

- Develop and continue improving your communication skills – writing, speaking. Take classes and ask for critiques. Join Toastmasters. Join your local chapter of the National Speakers Association.

- Be positive. It's good for your health, for that of your colleagues and for the organization.

- Be a lifelong learner. Think about interconnectedness and complexity. How can to connect your learning? How can you share what you've learned to add value?

- Be flexible and adaptable, ready to reestablish priorities in a changing environment.

- Don't take life — or yourself – too seriously. Have fun along the way.

The journey is the destination.

ACADEMIA

CHAPTER FOUR

Trying to Make the World a Better Place

by Ora Hirsch Pescovitz, MD

As early as I can remember, my parents taught me to make choices that leave the world in a better place. This philosophy drove me to be a physician and researcher. This is the philosophy by which my husband Mark and I raised our children. And this is the philosophy I follow – and share – as a leader. Making this world a better place in big and small ways is at the core of everything I do.

My love of research began in high school. When I was in ninth grade, I took a class called Research and Development. I was the only girl in the class, which I saw as a great advantage. During the first week of school, the teacher had us design a study using the scientific method. I decided to evaluate whether plants would grow better under the influence of classical music, the music of the Beatles or no music at all. Sadly, all of the plants died, which made it clear that I wasn't destined for a career in botany. However, the experience of investigation and the process of discovery—the fact that you could ask a question that hadn't been answered and design an experiment to investigate the question – ignited my passion for science and made me realize I wanted to dedicate my life to investigating questions that would result in ways to make sick people better. Although I didn't know the term at the time, that was the moment I decided to become a physician-scientist.

When I entered a six-year medical program in 1974, I was one of 15 women in a class of 60. Notably, today, women often make up half of incoming medical students. Again, as an 18-year-old college bound female, I saw this as advantageous-less dating competition! It was during my time in medical school that

I met my future husband, Mark Pescovitz.

When I was in Medical School, everyone said to me "of course you'll be a pediatrician because you're a girl and girls like children." Of course, this sexist assumption got right under my skin and caused me to vow that I would be anything BUT a pediatrician. And so I set out to become a surgeon.

Throughout my training, I fought every inclination toward pediatrics. I even went so far as to put off my required pediatrics rotation until the middle of my senior year. When I finally started that rotation, however, something unexpected and transformative happened: I found my vocation.

Upon completing medical school in 1979, Mark and I headed to the University of Minnesota where I completed my residency in pediatrics while he completed his residency in general surgery. From there, we moved to Maryland, where I completed my pediatrics residency at Children's Hospital National Medical Center in Washington, D.C., as well as a fellowship in endocrinology at the National Institutes of Health's Institute of Child Health and Human Development, while Mark did research training at the National Cancer Institute. During our time in the D.C. area, we welcomed our first two children – Aliza and Ari – who were born 16 months apart. Then, it was back to Minnesota for Mark to complete fellowships in transplantation and gastrointestinal endoscopy, while I served as an assistant professor of pediatric endocrinology and metabolism in the University of Minnesota's Department of Pediatrics. This was 1987, the same year we rounded out our family with the addition of our daughter, Naomi.

The following year was a bit of a crossroads for me. Mark and I received a number of offers for positions at various – but different – universities. Mark had been offered an assistant professorship in surgery at the Indiana University Medical Center – a position he very much wanted – but I wasn't offered an appealing position there. Also, I couldn't imagine living in Indianapolis! After much debate and discussion, we decided to let his career guide our next step, and the five of us were off to Indy.

The 21 years I spent in Indiana turned out to be ones that I treasure, both personally and professionally. I watched my three children evolve into wonderful adults; had the honor of treating many inspiring young patients at Riley Hospital for Children; and bolstered Indiana University's position as a focal point for biomedical research and a catalyst for Indiana's life sciences initiative.

Upon arriving in Hoosier country, I accepted an appointment as an associate professor of Pediatrics, and Physiology and Biophysics. Over the next several years, I began to establish myself within the IU community, becoming director of IU's section of Pediatric Endocrinology/Diabetology in 1990, the Edwin Letzter Professor of Pediatrics in 1998, executive dean for Research Affairs at IU School of Medicine from 2000-2009, president and CEO of Riley Hospital for Children from 2004-2009 and Interim Vice President for Research Administration from 2007-2009.

I spent 30 years of my career conducting basic and translational research in molecular endocrinology and treating children with growth and pubertal disorders. Pediatric endocrinology is a wonderful subspecialty because you have the opportunity to break down very complex issues and identify simplified solutions, as well as help children and families. One of my proudest accomplishments was co-authoring *Pediatric Endocrinology: Mechanisms and Management* with Dr. Erica Eugster.

In 2007, I experienced a serious career disappointment when I was one of two finalists for the presidency for Indiana University. I didn't get the job and my disappointment was palpable. I felt lost and unsure about my future for the very first time. But, sometimes you have to fail in order to win. And as the saying goes, when one door closes, another one opens.

When I decided to accept the position of Health System CEO and executive vice president for medical affairs at the University of Michigan in 2009, it was one of the most difficult decisions of my career. But, just like we did two decades before, Mark and I discussed the options and decided it was an opportunity I couldn't and shouldn't pass up. Our kids were all grown, Mark's career as a transplant surgeon was thriving and we decided that, like many dual-career couples, we would make it work. It was time for change and new opportunities, so off to Ann Arbor I went, and where I remain as I write this.

On leadership

It was only in the last few years that I took a turn on my career path and became involved in academic medical center administration. This change presented me with new challenges and opportunities to impact human health and the health care delivery system, while enabling me to remain closely connected to research, education and patient care. I describe my leadership style as what Robert Greenleaf calls "servant leadership." I am here to serve, and I believe that others in leadership roles are here to serve, as well. It's not about the leader; it's about the institution. A number of years ago, my career focused on my own research and taking care of patients. As I moved to more administrative roles, I realized that I had strengths in creating environments in which other people can thrive. It is very much like being a parent: You try to create an environment in which your children will be maximally nurtured so that one day they will eventually excel. In much the same way, as a leader, I am responsible for creating the environment in which those around me will thrive and be nurtured and the institution will be maximally successful.

As a physician, I learned how important it is to learn through observation. As a scientist, I know it's important to acquire data, be objective, let experiments tell the truth and not let your preconceived ideas sway you. As a hospital administrator, I've learned how important it is to be a member of a productive team. My leadership style is a culmination of these experiences, plus lessons learned through parenting.

I don't claim to be the smartest or most experienced person in the room. That's why I surround myself with experts and people who represent diverse perspectives. My job is to set the direction and vision, and make it safe for my team to be collegial collaborators and intelligent risk-takers. This can be tricky and difficult in health care, which traditionally is such a risk adverse industry. But, I encourage my team to take risks when it makes sense and to see failure as opportunity to learn and evolve.

Two final techniques that I have found to be critical factors in successful leadership are to create an environment that encourages and rewards creativity, and accept that you and others will make mistakes along the way – mistakes are invaluable learning opportunities. In fact, if you don't make mistakes along the way, you may not be trying hard enough!

On mentorship

To be successful and fulfilled, you should never stop learning, developing and growing personally or professionally, and mentors provide incredibly valuable guidance. I don't know if I would be where I am without mentors, and I don't think you can ever have too many of them. I don't think mentoring is emphasized and encouraged as much as it should be in today's world.

I've found that no one person can serve all your needs, so I have crafted what I like to call a "mentor quilt." A mentor quilt is a support network of inspiring individuals who serve as advisors for how you want to live both your personal and professional lives. I have one mentor for research, one for clinical, one for work-life balance and so on. I am always adding new ones – and I never let the others go. Find mentors, and be a mentor. I like the warmth and comfort that I experience when I wrap myself in the thoughts of my mentor quilt.

On work-life balance and time management

When my children were young, the approach of summer always meant more activities, which meant it was a good time for me to take a look at my own schedule and make sure that I could effectively be both Mom and doctor. While not always an easy task, it is certainly one of the most important.

Work-life balance is fundamental to our physical, mental and emotional wellness, as well as our productivity in – and satisfaction with – our professional and personal lives. In my experience, the key to balancing work and life effectively comes down to time management. I recall a proverb that says "Ordinary people think merely of spending time. Great people think of using it."

Over the course of my life and career, I've found that the best strategy for time management is following the Pareto Principle, or what is more commonly called the 80/20 Rule. Most things in life are distributed unevenly, including our "To Do" lists. Applying the 80/20 rule, typically 80% of the value from our work comes from only 20% of the items on our To Do lists. So, focus your energy and time on the 20% of tasks that result in 80% of the value – the ones that yield the greatest return on investment.

Of course, just invoking the name of Pareto won't make the less valuable 80% of tasks on your "To Do" list magically disappear. You need a strategy for managing those items, as well. One of the most successful strategies I've used is the 4Ds: Do; Dump; Delegate; Delay.

DO: This applies to those tasks that support your most valuable work – the vital 20%. Deal with e-mails, documents, phone calls regarding priority issues as soon as they come across your desk, your inbox or your voicemail. I call this "handle paper once." This way, you stay on top of your priorities, you keep important projects moving and you don't amass a daunting load to deal with at another time. That other time might be a long way off.

- DUMP: If something comes across your desk that doesn't pertain to your priorities, doesn't require follow up and doesn't support your goals, do you really need to keep it? Probably not—DUMP it!

- DELEGATE: If a task requires attention or action but doesn't make your "Do" list, can/should someone else handle it? Is it on another person's "Do" list? If so, move it along.

- DELAY: Very few things should make it to the Delay pile. But, on occasion, there may be something you want to review later.

If so, file, print or store it for another time.

Of course, there is no one-size-fits-all solution to time management or work-life balance. As our lives change, our priorities change and the balance we need changes, too. The 4Ds strategy has worked for me for many years, so I continue to use it. In fact, I revisit it almost daily to make sure I am on track. Find the formula and strategies that help you best use your time and achieve maximum work-life balance.

On the future of health care

The way we practice medicine and the business of health care are changing. Today, patients have more choices about where to get care and providers have more choices of where they refer their patients. At the same time, reimbursement to hospitals and physicians from insurance companies is becoming increasingly tied to quality and timeliness of care, as well as the overall patient experience. As competition for patients continues to escalate, health care organizations will need to further distinguish themselves or risk losing market share and clinical revenue. And as the consolidation of hospitals and practices continues, the business end of medicine is becoming even more important. We can't bury our heads in the sand.

As such, we have to become more nimble, more cost-effective, more adaptable, more collaborative, more globally-focused and just plain smarter. I find all of this very exciting! This is an incredible time to be in health care and to influence the evolution of medicine.

On happiness

Over the course of my career, I've noticed that successful people are almost always happy people. But, they are never content. If you let yourself be content, you welcome mediocrity into your life. If you are resting on your laurels, as Malcolm Kushner says, you are likely wearing them on the wrong end.
If, however, you find yourself in a place where you are just not happy with your job, I suggest trying out what I call the "4Ps":

> First, **P**ush and lobby for change that will change your circumstances.

> If that doesn't work, **P**ut up with it – accept the situation and decide to adapt to it.

> Still not working out? Well, it might be time to leave, or **P**ull

out. Sometimes leaving is the only way to move on and ahead.

And finally, no matter what, always find time to have fun, to enjoy life and to **P**lay.

On life and loss

On December 12, 2010, my life changed forever when my beloved husband, Mark, was killed in a tragic car accident. I thought my life was nearly perfect until his death.

Mark was a committed volunteer and leader in the Jewish art and music communities; a surgeon who always put patients first; a researcher determined to find new ways to save and improve lives; an artist who absorbed and reflected the world around him; and a dedicated father, husband, brother and son who embraced the true beauty and meaning of family. He was my soul mate, and now I am in the world without his love, companionship and friendship. Navigating the world without him is the most difficult thing I have ever had to do. But, the world does move on and I have begun that journey with amazing support from family and friends.

Mark's death reminded me about perspective. It re-grounded me and forced me to really connect to what is important and who I am. I can never replace him or replicate our life together, but I carry his wisdom and his love with me with every step forward. Life includes disappointments, tragedy, imperfections and heartache. It also includes amazing triumphs, discovery and great successes. Both offer you valuable opportunities to grow.

In a nutshell

Find a position in which you can maximize your strengths to make the greatest contribution.

- Cultivate an environment where people feel encouraged and rewarded for creativity.

- Throw fear out the window—take risks!!

- Embrace diversity in your colleagues and your organization.

- Realize that perfection is not success and failure is opportunity to learn and evolve.

- Accept that you will make mistakes. In fact, if you don't make mistakes along the way, you may not be trying hard enough!

- Find a suitable strategy for work-life balance. Work is important, but what else defines you?

- Create a "mentor quilt."

- Success breeds success, and leadership is about helping others succeed.

- Don't wait for opportunities to find you – seek them out and create them.

CHAPTER FIVE

Learning to Lead

by Donna Parker, MD

Perhaps people are born to lead, but many do not recognize that potential in themselves without others continuously pushing them to the front. My career has been a lot of being pushed to the front with a bit of asking to move forward sprinkled in. When I complete a "Myers-Briggs" self-assessment, I clearly fall into the category of a "leader." It's funny that I don't identify the constellation of character traits in myself which so clearly corresponds with those who like to lead.

Leadership has been defined as a process of social influence in which one person can enlist the aid and support of others in the accomplishment of a common task. What are those character traits? In no particular order, I think they are charisma, confidence, vision, interpersonal skills, vigor, enthusiasm, integrity, magnanimity and fairness. These are the parts of me that have allowed me to be a successful leader and role model in medicine.

I left high school in Maryland and went off to Canada for my undergraduate education at McGill University. I am often asked why I made that somewhat unusual choice. I guess it was a peek into my nature even at seventeen that I was a bit bold and confident with a good sense of adventure. I loved the idea of living in another country and especially living in a bilingual city. What an opportunity that was. McGill was a tremendous growth experience for me because of the diversity of the campus and the city. My French became quite good, and I met people whose families were from all parts of the world. The rigor of the academics kept me focused and engaged. I was a part of a very large student body, so I was able to remain rather anonymous, which if you ask me is the way I generally like it. My goal was to perform well and return to the United States to pursue medicine, and I did that.

I decided to attend the University of Maryland School of Medicine largely for geographical and financial reasons. It was time to move back closer to home, and as my state school it was economically appropriate. Perhaps if I had been thinking "leadership" then I might have courted the "higher profile" medical schools to augment my resume. However, I came to medical school with the hope of learning how to take care of patients without a real sense of what that meant over the course of a lifetime. I was the prototypical girl who was good in science class, so I was steered toward medicine. Because I enjoy social interactions, the thought that I could engage with patients was on target. But at the time I had no aspirations to be a leader in medical education.

The transition to Baltimore was a difficult one for me. I had left a very cosmopolitan, multicultural city for one which seemed to me to be stuck at least a decade in the past. Most of my classmates were from Baltimore, and a large number of them had attended regional colleges and universities. I was clearly an outsider. However, I did meet a lot of fun and interesting people in my class, and I remain friends with quite a few of them. A handful are still on the faculty at Maryland. About a third of my classmates were women. While we didn't feel particularly marginalized, there were still vestiges of earlier times with the locker rooms in the OR at one local hospital labeled "doctors" and "nurses." We tended to laugh rather than become angry.

While medical school was intellectually fascinating, it was sometimes clinically harsh with tired residents and attendings not always seeming to truly care for or about patients. I found only a few people I would consider role models or mentors, and that concerned me. Had I made the right career choice? Clinical medicine was a theoretical good match, but would it be in practice? Were there other options I should be considering? The enthusiasm for my chosen work was not there. Through all of these questions, my mentors remained very supportive and over the ensuing years provided consistent advice and encouragement.

I was sent adrift into an internal medicine residency hoping for a spark. In the long hours, days and weeks of residency, I learned that I enjoyed the fast pace and quick decision making required when working in the ICU and in the outpatient clinic. In both of these areas, I also appreciated working collaboratively with staff to solve patient care problems. There was great satisfaction in seeing patients' lives changed in the moment in the ICU and over time in the clinic. I was easily engaged by patients' stories about who they were and how they led their lives. So, there was a place for me in clinical medicine. I just had to find the right situation. I was developing a vision for my future.

Adrift again, moving with my husband to North Carolina where he was beginning a fellowship, I had no job and continuing uncertainty about what sort of career suited me. I eventually secured a position at Wake Medical Center in Raleigh which was a University of North Carolina affiliate with medical students and residents rotating in both inpatient and outpatient areas. The position afforded me a lot of primary patient care responsibility along with a significant role in the training of the medical students and residents. It seemed like an ideal first job out of residency.

Having once again been bold, picking up and moving to a new place with a new culture and values, I learned much about people and the art of medicine. I grew exponentially as a clinician by sheer volume and diversity of patient issues. HIV was just emerging as an entity, and I experienced both the pain and reward of caring for young gay men who had left North Carolina for more tolerant places, but were obligated by circumstances to return home to die. Because of the vigor with which I approached my work, I was asked to co-manage the outpatient clinic and to coordinate our portion of the UNC physical diagnosis course for medical students. I also saw a need for organized pre-operative evaluations for patients at our site and started a clinic for that purpose. Looking back on this time, I enjoyed the spirit of the students, the constant learning through educating and creating order out of chaos. These have remained ongoing themes in my career since that time.

Recognizing where I found joy, as we were moving back to Baltimore to be near family, I began looking for a position that involved both working with learners and administrative responsibilities. As fate would have it, the position of Director of Medical Clinic was open at the University of Maryland School of Medicine (UMSoM). Fortunately, I'd been a good student with strong interpersonal skills, so no bridges had been burned and people with whom I'd worked as a student were still there to recommend my hire. I must admit it was a little uncomfortable stepping into a new system and being immediately in charge. However, if handled well, those situations can be the source of much personal growth. I was very keen about the prospect of mentoring the internal medicine residents in their outpatient experience and felt I could develop a vision for making their experience better.

During this time, I learned that it is important to really understand current systems before implementing changes and to carefully assess what works well and what does not. The next step is to figure out who has power to make necessary changes if that person is not you. I diligently kept abreast of policies, procedures and curricula at other programs to incorporate new ideas. I attended national meetings to meet others in like positions. The Internal Medicine Program Director eventually asked me to coordinate all of the outpatient education for the residents and to develop an ambulatory block rotation curriculum. Upon completion of that task, I asked for a promotion based upon my expanded duties and the structure of departmental education at other programs. That's how I became the Director of Ambulatory Education. I believe if I hadn't asked for a different title, it would not have been offered. So lesson learned: a little push can help to advance your career.

Concurrent with my return to UMSoM, the Admissions Committee was expanding in size. I volunteered to join in order to increase my knowledge of the medical school administration and to participate in a process I considered quite meaningful. The Associate Dean had known me as a medical student, and I believe that facilitated the acceptance of a new faculty member. My diligent work, punctuality and full engagement at meetings were recognized, and the Associate Dean also valued my integrity and fairness in thinking through situations that arose.

All of this led to an offer to be Assistant Dean a year later. This position was my first real foot in the door as a medical school administrator. I served in the Admissions Office and on the Admissions Committee for 13 years. I learned everything I could about the policies and processes of the office even though on paper it was just 10 percent of my time. Putting added effort into something about which you are passionate is the lesson here. The reward is the chance to spend more of your time doing those types of activities in future positions.

At this point, I had also reached the time in my life when I wanted to start a family. Trying to simultaneously begin an academic career created some challenges and surprises. Up to now, pursuit of a career was all I had ever known. I had never considered working less than full time, but while on maternity leave with my first child, it became quite clear that I couldn't be both the physician/educator and the mother I wanted to be with a full-time position. My colleagues warned me that the Department of Medicine had never signed off on a part-time faculty member and attempting to be the first would be folly. Because I was so certain of my decision, I was prepared to look for a new job should my request be denied. Fortunately, after explaining that I could accomplish the important tasks working part-time, the Department agreed.

Many people will tell you that working part-time means full-time work with part-time pay, and there is definitely some truth in that. But for me, the biggest advantage was flexibility in my schedule. Although I cut back by giving up one of my two patient sessions each week and my inpatient attending work, I was able to do the rest of the work in the hours that suited my family. Being part-time meant no one harassed me for leaving at 3:30 to get to a lacrosse game. That alone was worth it to me, and I was lucky to have the financial resources to handle the decrement in pay. My physician husband had a terrific job that could certainly cover our expenses if I needed a bit of time off before seeking part-time work that would accommodate motherhood. He was an important part of the decision making to devote more time than initially planned to our growing family. We now have two children, and I have been working part-time for 18 years with gradually increasing work hours from 60 percent to 80 percent. I plan to transition back to full-time work as our oldest daughter heads off to college this fall and the younger one acquires her driver's license. Hopefully, this will be a smooth and positive transition.

The next twist in my career came about seven years after joining the faculty when I accepted an offer to become the Associate Dean for Student and Faculty Development. This was a newly created office, and that scenario presented both opportunity and challenges. I was initially offered the position at the As-sistant Dean level, which would have represented a lateral move from a job I loved. I held out for the Associate Dean position with increased autonomy and the prospect of defining a new office. The fact that I would be supervising two staff members meant that I would acquire more skills managing people and budgets. There were also a few existing education grants which had been handled by an office folded into this new one, so I had to quickly learn how to manage those. I created a faculty development curriculum and recruited fac-ulty members to participate in teaching workshops and small group sessions. The advising system for our medical students had also eroded, so I worked to create a new one, pairing a student and faculty member based upon similar interests (academic, personal or both).

The Student and Faculty Development office was successful in many areas, but I never felt it really had a defined identity. Ultimately, it was bits and pieces of lots of programs. Looking back, I am grateful for having learned more about personnel management, budgets and grants. However, I didn't love the work and was probably ready for another change after a few years.

It took six years before I was offered the position of Associate Dean for Student Affairs with larger staff and more responsibility. My acceptance actually required quite a bit of pushing because the Office of Student Affairs (OSA) had a number of active issues that needed to be addressed in short order. I was also in the final stages of pursuing a new education grant with site visitors arriving imminently. I understood that the path to promotion within the medical school was through grant and journal article writing, and that the move to OSA would likely put those activities on hold for a number of years, if not forever. Ultimately, I accepted the position because I felt that I had the organizational and leadership skills needed to substantially improve the office, and I truly cared about the education and well-being of our medical students. I set aside the immediate goal of promotion and moved to the position which I felt would provide greater personal rewards.

In retrospect, I believe I made the correct decision. Students who graduated prior to my move have returned to the OSA and are amazed at the changes. Much of my success is attributable to hiring the right people to work with me. As a condition of taking the position, I requested the hire of an additional Assistant Dean of my choosing at 40 percent effort. He has been amazing. As other faculty who'd been working in the office retired or moved on, I have hired three more Assistant Deans, two of whom are still in OSA. I aim to be magnanimous in my praise of their work and always try to do more than my fair share of all of the duties within the office. Our camaraderie and teamwork is the situation others dream of, and I feel very fortunate to have all of them around. We make each other better.

The greatest lesson I have learned as I move up in management roles in academia, is to never be afraid to take the lead if in your heart you know you have something to contribute and the skills to move others forward with you. I cannot say that I know where my career will take me over the next decade, but I imagine that I will remain engaged in activities related to undergraduate medical education since that is where I find joy. In all endeavors, it is important to remain open to new opportunities, to continue to learn and grow academically and personally and to follow your passion always.

HOSPITALS

CHAPTER SIX

Female Physicians as Hospital Administrators

by Kathleen Yaremchuk, MD, MSA

When I finished medical school and began residency, it never crossed my mind to consider the cost of the tests I ordered for my patients. As a physician, I believed my sole responsibility was to take care of the patient. It was the "administration's" job to keep the lights burning and deal with the financial aspects of running a hospital.

My career began as a general surgical intern at Cook County Hospital in Chicago, caring for the city's uninsured, where physicians were not concerned with costs of care or the financial aspects of the hospital. I don't think I ever saw an administrator during my tenure. The same was true as an otolaryngology resident at the University of Chicago. Although some patients were insured, we took care of everyone in the Emergency Department including victims of the "Gun and Knife Club of the South Side of Chicago." During rounds or when seeing uninsured patients in clinic, the cost of recommended procedures or the possible turning out of the patient who couldn't pay was not discussed. The "paperwork" under my purview then usually consisted of surgery consent and operating room (OR) forms required to board a case.

Following residency, I became a contract physician for the Great Lakes Naval Hospital in Illinois. With military salaries relatively low compared to private or academic practice physicians, the Navy had difficulty recruiting and keeping specialty physicians. I was hired by a physician group in Texas that provided specialty coverage for the military throughout the United States. Once again, I was in an environment that shunned discussion of costs or reimbursement since this was a single payer system covering all health care needs of military retirees, active duty personnel and their family members.

About this time, the national dialogue started on the rising cost of health care in the United States. I became interested in learning more about the infrastructure of hospital administration and researched available degree programs. In 1982, Northwestern University and the University of Chicago offered executive Master Degree programs in hospital administration, so I decided to apply to both. When I received the applications and request for college transcripts and Graduate Management Aptitude Test (GMAT) scores, I recognized how different the academic structures were between business schools and postgraduate training of medical school and residency. The GMAT covered topics far removed from my studies of gross anatomy, physiology, and surgery. To prepare for the GMAT, I enrolled in a review course like other prospective graduate business students.

I was ecstatic when my GMAT results scored in the 94th percentile. With a transcript from the University of Michigan's accelerated 6-year Integrated Premedical-Medical Program, I felt confident that I would be accepted at both schools. My only worry was how to decide which program would best serve my future endeavors. Imagine my surprise when not one but both schools rejected my application. Apparently an application from someone with a Medical Degree in 1982 was so unusual that Business School Admissions offices had no idea how to evaluate the application. I had no recent classes in economics, social studies, or English literature, which was the norm for their other applicants. The fact that an individual in the top 5 percent of college graduates who had graduated from medical school was more than likely to successfully complete any graduate degree program was not considered.

In 1984, I was recruited by Henry Ford Hospital in Detroit as an otolaryngologist. I had spent my clinical years there during medical school and enjoyed the large multispecialty group practice atmosphere. The Henry Ford Medical Group provided clinical care in the city and suburbs while maintaining an academic mission and commitment to the triad of patient care, education, and research. Shortly after my arrival at Henry Ford I was appointed Division Head of Otolaryngology at the satellite clinic where I practiced. I hadn't thought much about the title and was actually amused when a secretary congratulated me on the appointment. The division consisted of two half-time otolaryngologists and me. I didn't feel there was much to manage so the title seemed somewhat meaningless. What I failed to appreciate was that in addition to the otolaryngologists, there were audiologists, medical assistants, clinical service representatives, and hearing aid technicians for whom I was now responsible.

This position allowed me to participate in monthly division head meetings of all clinical departments. The forum discussed management issues and changes occurring within the Henry Ford Medical Group, and gave me exposure to the leadership of the satellite medical center as well as an opportunity to join other committees. By practicing at the site, I established my clinical credibility with patients and other providers. I believe it is imperative for a medical leader to have a strong, positive reputation in their field of clinical practice. The commitment to patients and clinical expertise is used as an indicator of commitment to the institution and its mission. Time and again, my reputation as a clinician has been a guiding force in my administrative success.

The Henry Ford Hospital began in 1915 when Henry Ford bought the hospital from the city of Detroit for one dollar. The city administration lacked funds to complete the hospital and was glad to have the industrialist take it off of their hands. Mr. Ford visited Johns Hopkins and the Mayo Clinic to better understand how to proceed with his vision of "the best hospital the city has seen". He readily acknowledged his lack of experience in building or running a hospital. He found he liked the multispecialty group practice clinic model of the Mayo Clinic and admired the educational rigor of Johns Hopkins, so he hired a surgeon from Johns Hopkins to become the first Chief of Staff of Henry Ford Hospital. The multispecialty group practice built then is now the Henry Ford Medical Group with more than 1,200 physicians.

When I joined Henry Ford in 1984, the group employed 350 physicians and an equal number of residents and fellows. In metropolitan Detroit, the Henry Ford Medical Group pioneered the development of suburban ambulatory clinics that would provide care and direct admissions to the 900-bed tertiary care Henry Ford Hospital within the city. Over time, an integrated delivery system developed, evolving into the Henry Ford Health System with acquisitions of an insurance company, several suburban hospitals, existing group practices, nursing homes, and home health care providers.

For me, this growth provided exposure to areas of health care delivery different from my experience as a clinician. Moreover, a large organization like the Henry Ford Health System was able to offer its employees various educational opportunities. In an employee newsletter, I discovered that Central Michigan University (CMU) offered a Master of Science in Administration (MSA) program with a core curriculum similar to postgraduate education in hospital administration. Meanwhile, our medical group's Board of Governors decided that a key strategy for future success was to develop a career path for physician leaders with an associated educational process. I was halfway through the MSA at CMU when word of my participation in the program reached the

Chief Medical Officer of our medical group. I was invited to chair the Physicians Leadership Development Council, giving me access to all physicians in our large medical group who were interested in Medical Management.

Concurrently, my responsibilities as Division Head in Otolaryngology-Head & Neck Surgery grew as I demonstrated competence in the role of an administrator. I was named Medical Director for Specialty Services at the satellite medical center where I practiced. This gave me responsibility for 14 medical and specialty divisions and the ambulatory surgery center. I determined salaries, oversaw performance reviews, budget development, and implementation of new programs in a collaborative, matrix management process with the chairs of the academic departments. I thrived on improving services and solving problems. It was important to involve physicians in their practice and have them understand how to balance the budget.

There couldn't have been a better place for me than Henry Ford Health System. The concept of a vertically integrated health system that was being discussed nationally was actually being built in Detroit.

After nine years of managing physicians, an opportunity arose as part of a joint venture with Henry Ford to become Vice President of Medical Affairs (VPMA) at a 268-bed hospital in an impoverished area of Detroit. Here was a chance for on-the-job training in hospital administration. In this role I also served as Medical Director for five primary care clinics. The hospital and primary care clinics faced the typical daunting problems associated with an inner city including poverty, poor health status, high unemployment, and safety from crime. The patient population served was largely Medicaid and Medicare with financial losses of $18 million the year I assumed the position.

As VP, I was responsible for hospital activities such as credentialing, utilization management, quality assurance and Joint Commission for Accreditation of Healthcare Organization (JCAHO) standards. The ambulatory clinics had 250,000 patient visits annually and a budget of $10 million. Like many, I believe that problems can be opportunities. I regarded the problems here as potential learning opportunities. Moreover, I knew that by successfully solving these problems, my reputation as a "change agent" would be set.

The medical staff at the hospital was composed of minority and international graduates. Some questioned how a white female surgical specialist from the suburbs would fit into such a diverse environment. The title of VPMA did not ensure acceptance by the medical staff. I knew I would have to "walk the talk" to make converts. My predecessors had been full-time administrators who never admitted or treated patients, so they were viewed with mistrust.

I made it a point to conduct a clinic in the hospital, operate on patients, and take call for emergencies. This gave me access to the emergency department, operating rooms (OR), and hospital inpatient units. These are places where poor management and performance can cause exceptionally large problems in a hospital. It did not take long for the grapevine to convey that I was a working VP. Influential members of the medical staff would talk to me on the inpatient units or in the OR lounge. If anything earns respect in a hospital, it is working shoulder to shoulder with the medical staff.

Over the course of two years, I learned about the politics of community hospitals and the issues of building a committed medical staff. I sought small victories by looking into areas with little or no resistance to change. Critical pathways were introduced to the hospital by being a champion and discussing the subject with those influential physicians with whom I had built relationships.

Much like the military, it is difficult to recruit needed specialists to an urban facility. I discovered that the only neurologist on staff who would see our ambulatory patients was writing unnecessary prescriptions for narcotics. Then he would ask the patients to return to his office after getting their medication at the pharmacy, ostensibly to make sure the prescription had been filled correctly. He would find an "error" and take the drugs from the patient. Since the patients did not pay for their medications, they were thankful for the so-called oversight. A nurse in my clinic tipped me to the scheme, and after an investigation I had to terminate the physician.

Another unfortunate experience involved a physician with the highest volume admissions to the hospital. As the physician for multiple nursing homes, he would admit patients to our hospital, but never round on them, instead allowing his nurse to direct their care. After documenting this physician's inappropriate care and charting irregularities, I suggested that the hospital CEO terminate his privileges. Unfortunately, that didn't happen and, as a result, I resigned from my position. When I received a call from the FBI and later read that this physician had been convicted of Medicare fraud, I knew that my education in hospital administration was complete.

Although ethically I had done what was right, raising that red flag ultimately caused problems in my career advancement. For several years afterward, my career stalled. I applied for positions and was never selected. I finally asked for an interview with the Chief Medical Officer. Although the meeting was cordial, it was clear that there were "issues". It was an educational experience because I learned that by rocking the boat, I now had "baggage". I was perceived as a "difficult" person to work with.

From that meeting, it was clear I needed to reinvent myself within the institution. I found an opportunity as a Medical Director for an insurance company owned by Henry Ford Health System. It was a great position that allowed me to continue my clinical work while earning credits in "Insurance 101". I was introduced into the process of concurrent review for inpatients, prior authorization of procedures, and medical necessity versus patient preference.

Through concurrent review, I recognized that most hospitals function five days a week, yet charge the same inpatient rates for seven days a week. Most interventions occur during week days. Patients admitted toward the end of the week usually had to wait over the weekend for their procedures. The irony is that they are too ill to go home, but well enough to wait a few days for a necessary procedure. In my view, it seems that hospitals should charge, and insurance companies should pay, different rates for weekdays versus weekends.

The process of prior authorization was another eye opener. I would request a physician's records to determine the evaluation that preceded the decision to perform a procedure and receive a one word illegible note from the physician with a medical assistant's assessment of the chief complaint. I was surprised that the physician would charge for an office visit with such cursory office notes.

It was also apparent that direct consumer advertising for procedures and medications was driving up the cost of care. When a maternity patient wanted an "under water delivery" that she'd heard was better for the newborn , she demanded an out-of-state referral. My response was a resounding denial of the request. While the consumer may feel that the delivery of her newborn into a whirlpool bath is a kinder way to come into this world, that is "patient preference," not "medical necessity".

As an active member of the Academy of Otolaryngology-Head and Neck Surgery (AAO-HNS), I had the opportunity to be appointed to the National Committee for Quality Assurance (NCQA) Practicing Physician Advisory Committee. This introduced me to the world of quality in health care - probably the single best use of my time with payback in ways I never could have imagined. Several times a year in my role as physician surveyor for NCQA and member of the Review Oversight Committee, I traveled to health plans around the country evaluating their performance on quality and service - two important areas in health care. My time with NCQA helped me in my Otolaryngology roles. I recently received a national award from the AAO-HNS for my community service associated with quality and have been named chair of the Advisory Council of Quality for the AAO/HNS.

My expanded experience in insurance, quality, and clinical care also helped me grow within the Henry Ford Health System. I became involved in the pay-for-performance insurance movement and Centers of Excellence designations. Within the Henry Ford Medical Group, I became the knowledge expert and negotiated with insurance companies and submitted applications to regulatory agencies. Success begets success as I was recognized as someone with a unique skill set. Added to my role then as Vice Chair of the Department of Otolaryngology in the medical group, I became Vice President for Clinical Practice Performance for the health system. This new VP title was actually one that I created to reflect the combination of quality metrics and cost effectiveness that payers were evaluating. It was a bold move to develop a position and job description for something that never before existed. Acceptance of my proposal by the Chief Medical Officer of the medical group was a significant learning moment: Look at who you want to be and what you want to do, and the rest is history!

Some suggest that I continue to take on "titles" and am involved in more things than most people can remember. I regard this as my continuing education process. In each new role I give what I have gleaned from every past position and continue to learn more. Nothing in life stands still, so as an individual, an administrator, or a physician, we need to continue to grow, changing what we do to stay relevant and provide a unique service.

I had never considered my future to be a Chair of a department. In 2008, after our Otolaryngology chief moved to another institution, a search committee appointed by the Chief Medical Officer and Executive Vice President of the Henry Ford Medical Group was set up to choose the next chairperson. I was suddenly faced with the dilemma of applying for the chair position or watching someone else assume the role. Ultimately, I submitted my letter of interest along with 14 applicants from around the country. I wanted the most competent individual for the position to be selected, and while I hoped to be the committee's choice, I decided that whomever they selected would be appropriate.

During the selection process, I was appointed interim chair for Otolaryngology. I moved to the "corner office" and dealt with issues of the department while also serving in my role as Vice Chair of Clinical Practice Performance and practicing clinically. After a year, I was officially offered the position of Chair of the Department of Otolaryngology-Head & Neck Surgery at Henry Ford Hospital. When I assumed the role, we had six otolaryngologists in the department. Three years later I have hired eight new otolaryngologists.

An urban legend suggests that it is impossible to recruit professionals to Detroit because of its poor economic climate and bad reputation. Obviously, to recruit new otolaryngologists willing to commit their professional careers to the institution, the draw must be a world class department. In the beginning, someone likened my tenacious recruiting efforts to that of a "rabid bulldog". But my persistence paid off. I now have people sending me their curriculum vitae's and approaching me for positions.

Of the 103 Otolaryngology-Head and Neck Surgery academic departments or departments with residency positions, there are only four female department chairs. When I finished residency in 1982, 98.5 percent of the specialty was male. Currently 50 percent of medical students are female and the number of female residents is increasing. There is still a glass ceiling within the specialty for females; the dilutional effect of moving from 98.5 percent of otolaryngologists being male to a 50:50 ratio will take years. I joke that we can still meet in a sedan and don't need an SUV to seat a quorum.

When we interview medical students for residency positions it is an interesting dynamic. I believe a disproportionate number of females submit applications to our institution because we have a female chair and three of 12 senior staff physicians are females.

As I recruit new residents and staff, I am committed to making each one a "star" within our specialty. My job is to help them be as successful as possible while furthering the reputation and goals of the department. It is a win-win from my perspective.

Similarly, the national reputation of the Department has grown. I explain our success in basketball terms. If Le Bron James is the only star playing on your team, the team can only go so far. On the other hand, if you have a team of talented individuals without superstar status like the Detroit Pistons, you can become NBA champions. My goal as department chair is to emulate the Detroit Pistons approach. I am not the star of my team. Rather, I coach and support talented individuals to create a team of champions.

Recently our health system, hospitals, and medical group have focused on succession planning for executive leadership positions. They want to be prepared as natural turnover occurs and leaders reach retirement. I have been selected as one of two internal candidates for such an executive position. This has created yet another dilemma since the role would require my moving on from my current position as chair of Otolaryngology.

Coincidentally, I was also asked to be Chair of the Operations Council for our medical group. This Council did not previously exist, so I have been wading into uncharted waters. Rather than waiting for someone to tell me "no", I decided to write its destiny by taking on any challenge to our medical group that could be considered "operational". It may be a bold approach, but I've learned that nature abhors a vacuum. If no one else is performing the function, it is fair game to take control, make changes, and see what happens.

Outside of my health system, I receive offers for Otolaryngology-Head and Neck Surgery positions and as well as Chief Medical Officer jobs. In which direction I will go is an open question. The key factor in making my decision for my next professional role will be to find the greatest opportunity for future development and progress. It is important to be passionate about your work. It's equally important to be able to invigorate those around you to do the best that they can. I am now in the mentoring mode for women of all clinical specialties within my institution. I am also mentoring women within otolaryngology to assume Chair positions.

Lessons Learned

A prime lesson in the field of medicine is to develop a passion for a particular area of clinical medicine and medical management, and accept all opportunities to learn. You never know where these paths lead. Most important, to build a positive reputation means to do the work, show up for meetings, contribute to discussions, and volunteer for assignments. Combining present knowledge with future learning will only add to your leadership skills.

I have also learned that others' perceptions of you can make or break your future career advancement. If this happens or you seem to have reached a "dead end" in your career, figure out a way to add new tools to your toolbox and then move forward. There are always new concepts and analytic approaches to dealing with the healthcare system. By keeping yourself on the cutting edge, not only will there be opportunities to make yourself invaluable to your own institution, but to other healthcare organizations as well.

Finally, it is important to communicate your goals. The meeting before the meeting is the most important groundwork that can be laid to assure success.

Personally, I have raised three children, the youngest of whom just left for his first year of college. The children were present when I received an endowed chair from Henry Ford Health System and the national award from the AAO/HNS. They recognize my contribution to medicine and are proud of their mother. After 33 years of marriage I was recently divorced, but I can assure you it was not because I chose a career over my marriage. Looking back, I would not have done anything differently.

There is no question in my mind that physicians are uniquely positioned to lead health care reform and function as health care administrations at any level. Open the door and walk through the executive suite of your hospital or organization without fear. You belong there.

CHAPTER SEVEN

Knowledge is Power: A Journey of Transition

by Eneida O. Roldan, MD, MPH, MBA

"You make a living by what you get. You make a life by what you give"

— *Winston Churchill*

The drive to know more, give more and make a difference has been my primary motivator in both my professional and personal life. Since childhood, I was inquisitive, always thinking outside the box. I refused to accept the status quo on any matter that came my way. Although my ways were often unpopular and uncomfortable to the mainstream, the overriding quest for knowledge made it all worthwhile.

In this chapter, I share my journey into the world of Medical Management. That journey focuses on the value I place as an executive on soft skills (also called Emotional Intelligence). These have helped me master challenging career transitions by increasing self-awareness, knowing the best "fit" for my talents, keeping a positive attitude, embracing change and finally overcoming adversity.

All of these skills have ultimately helped my personal growth. You will not find a guide on how I became an executive using hard skills here. I assume those physicians/professionals reading this have mastered those skills through many years of schooling. This chapter will document my personal journey. While it may seem unconventional, there are lessons for anyone transitioning from clinician to physician leadership roles.

My career in medical management really began in childhood. As my first mentor, my maternal grandmother taught me never to accept the status quo. Although I didn't know then that someday I would make the transition from a "white coat" to a "suit", her early lessons became the core for my belief that any successful transition or change in life is a choice. That choice should be made with a foundation of purpose to better who you are or want to become; with direction that has both conviction and support from others including mentors and family; and with a clear focus on goals while staying true to your values, never compromising integrity, honesty, or ethics. This has played a major role in my journey. Change is inevitable. It is how you deal with it—the loss of the known to an unknown—including the chaos of transition—that makes you successful. I knew I wanted to go to medical school at the age of eight. I was inquisitive, always seeking answers and interested in how the human body works. I graduated from medical school and entered the most basic science specialty, Pathology. Colleagues and mentors alike asked why I chose that field. They told me I was a "people person" and that Pathologists worked away from people, behind the scenes. Facing this stereotyping/status quo challenged me to teach those questioning my choice that it is far too easy to think inside the box. If I had then, I would have missed a wonderful opportunity.

Much to my surprise, Pathology offered a great foundation for a career in management. It taught me to work in teams and that technology has an important role in medicine. It also provided the opportunity to learn to budget an organization. Running a lab is all about knowing how to implement quality standards for products and services, working as part of interdisciplinary teams, and producing a product with the highest standards at an affordable price. I didn't choose Pathology knowing this would be a great field to acquire the knowledge that would help me as a medical manager. I simply chose the specialty that satisfied my quest to learn the origin of disease processes and mechanisms in depth.

During my residency program, I was fortunate to find another mentor. She was a faculty member and the Director of the Department of Pediatric Pathology. She taught me that without passion there can be no progress in your life's endeavors—either personal or professional. Passion allows you to share talents, while complacency and apathy constrains progress and growth. Passion opens your world to new ideas and enables you to accept change with an open mind. Her words embodied the role passion can play in different aspects of the journey. It is with both passion and self-awareness that we begin to understand who we are, where we are going, and if we even like our direction.

My mantra became: "In the face of change, conviction, purpose and passion provide the drive to accept a transition in pursuit of a different direction and opportunities." I vowed to be open for any opportunity that would nurture passion, fulfill a purpose, and represent a positive change of direction. I also focused on nurturing my soft skills (Emotional Intelligence).

The healthcare system today is going through tremendous transitions. These changes have already begun to affect the practicing physician's role. This has created chaos in the status quo world of the physician/clinician. After spending so much of their lives studying and competing to be the best in their medical school class and their specialty field, some have expressed doubt about their future value as medical doctors. Faced with the reality of this transition, they are afraid of change. However, for those who already have or can acquire the needed skills and want to play a part in the evolution of a new healthcare delivery system as leaders, there are tremendous opportunities.

Despite the increase in the number of physician executives, I believe that most are still not viewed as great managers. In the minds of many—including some physicians themselves—doctors should just treat patients. After all, the argument goes, that's why they went to medical school. I don't agree. Physicians embody hard work, dedication, and commitment which make them perfect candidates to face the challenges of any transition they may encounter or consciously choose. As I learned from my grandmother/mentor, it is how the transition and willingness to change is handled that will lead to a successful outcome.

Women physician executives face the same or greater challenges than those they have encountered as female clinicians. This is especially true as more women continue to climb the corporate ladder to the C-suite. The key is to use the skills necessary to overcome adversity in the face of transition. I will personally share those that have and continue to work for me, with the proviso that everyone needs to learn which skills successfully work for them.

In every journey, we encounter opportunities. What's important is to have the proper foundation to recognize them and be ready to seize them. After having been successful in private practice for twelve years, I decided to pursue formal education in Public Health and entered a Masters program focused on developing public health programs. This provided an opportunity to engage in population-based medicine and, more importantly, to learn how to make these programs administratively and operationally successful. After graduation, I realized I needed more formal financial acumen, so I enrolled in a physician executive MBA program.

This turned out to be the best decision I made in my transition to administrative medicine. As my network grew inside and outside of medicine, business world contacts called to engage me on projects integrating medicine and business. I was suddenly learning business firsthand. One of my earliest projects was for a group of entrepreneurs who needed a physician with business knowledge—someone who could speak the business lingo while integrating concepts of medicine into business. From this experience, I learned "speed to market" and "Carpe diem" (seize the day) as well as concepts that I currently use in my new endeavor. I was well on my journey of transition.

Subsequently, I was offered the role of President and CEO for a local community hospital that had recently filed for bankruptcy protection. Located in Miami, Florida, the facility was the first Hispanic hospital opened in the city at the beginning of the Cuban exile in 1963. Every important Cuban community leader had some personal connection to it. Being of Cuban decent myself, I was especially passionate about wanting to do my part to save the hospital. At the same time, I was aware that if the outcome was not positive, I might not be able to remain in the Miami area and pursue a career in hospital administration. Staying true to my mantra, I accepted the job which turned out to be an incredible learning experience. The Board and I ultimately transitioned the hospital out of bankruptcy and sold it, thus preventing closure and the loss of services to that community.

As a result of this success, the local community came to view me as a capable administrator. After passing the gavel on to the new President and CEO of the community hospital, I realized I wanted a greater challenge. Never did I imagine that I would be asked to join Jackson Health System as the Administrator of their flagship hospital, Jackson Memorial Hospital. This was the same medical center where I had studied and become a trained physician.

This became another journey of passion as well as the chance to use both hard and soft skills for the betterment of many. To be able to serve the place that made my physician journey a reality was truly a wonderful opportunity. But not everything that shines is gold. There are many who agree that I took on one of the hardest jobs in the country, not only because of the extraordinary challenges that are part and parcel of any ailing hospital system, but because as the appointed "savior" of a public organization, I had to juggle city/county/ state politics while trying to focus on my purpose.

Within the first eight months of my tenure, the President and CEO of the Jackson Health System announced his departure. I was seen as the heir apparent. Once again, I faced another change in direction. I had to make a decision as to whether or not I would consider the role of President and CEO of the entire system. After much thought, but with a continued desire to grow by challenging myself, I decided to announce my candidacy. This decision resulted in the most challenging and eye-opening experiences along my career path.

Jackson Health System is both a public health system and an academic medical center. It is one of the largest public health systems in the country and the largest in the state of Florida. Its funding depends on public dollars, local economy and hospital operations. Unfortunately, my announced candidacy and subsequent confirmation coincided with unprecedented flux in healthcare and a serious downturn in our country's economy.

The challenges I faced in this role would mold the rest of journey. The most important and difficult lesson I learned was that my values were not aligned with the values of those in power. Once that became clear, I came face to face with a dilemma familiar to many administrators: what to do when personal ethics conflict with policies and politics of those who have ultimate control? In my case I clashed with the governing board—The Public Health Trust—and the Miami Dade County Commission. As difficult as it was to acknowledge, I had to accept the fact that ultimately my own direction had to change. I decided not to renew my contract.

After that experience, I made a conscious decision to choose organizations where my "fit" would serve a purpose. In this phase of my career, I wanted to own a piece of what I could create. I am currently the Chief Executive Officer of a start-up company focusing on telehealth—an area in which I believe I can provide solutions to many of the problems within the healthcare delivery system. This opportunity offers flexibility, innovation, integration of all my skills (medicine, administration, and network) and a huge potential for growth. It also enables me to continue teaching at the College of Medicine—an important part of my transition decision. I want to share my given talents. I know this new role will not be free of challenges or problems. Nevertheless, having the tools to face them and the ability to accept transition will make any change more bearable.

As I wrote at the start of this chapter, developing soft skills/emotional intelligence was key to my successful journey from pathologist to physician executive. These skills have helped me develop self-awareness, sharpen my decision-making skills, and learn to accept transition with a positive attitude. They have also helped me deal with the psychological and emotional strain that is part of leaving the status quo, a place of comfort. Implementing these skills has enabled me to have an open mind to recognize and seize great opportunities. Each of these opportunities has expanded my knowledge base, giving me power to be successful.

Finally, the balance of work and family is important to complete a successful journey. Being the wife of a surgeon and the mother of three, I know this all too well. It is very lonely at the top. A family bond built on unconditional love and support along with my faith has kept me grounded and given me the strength to continue to face challenges. Maintaining an open dialogue with my husband and children and prioritizing tasks allowed me to continue moving along my career path. I could share my doubts, my weaknesses, my difficulties openly without fear of rejection. That gave me the energy, courage, and hope needed to face another day.

Despite the fact that there is more acceptance of women in management today, the issue of balancing work and family is, unfortunately, still primarily a woman's issue. As a physician executive, there will be times when family may suffer for the sake of work and vice versa. Having a supportive family will provide the wherewithal to face any adversity.

At this point in time, physicians have the opportunity to take the lead role in changing how healthcare is delivered. Those entering the world of management have an important role to fill. I believe physicians—women and men—are the best equipped to manage change in healthcare. Below are some bullet points that summarize my advice to those physicians who wish to become successful in the world of medical management. This is a world that may not be comfortable at first, but in which there is much to gain, personally and professionally.

- **Keep passion in all your pursuits.**

- **Never shortchange your quest for knowledge. Formal education and experience are key to success.**

- **Never accept the status quo even if it means going against the mainstream.**

- **Keep your values firmly grounded and never compromise them. It isn't worth it.**

- **Learn from others. There are many mentors. Grow your network.**

- **Keep your options open. Every opportunity is a learning experience. Choose the right "fit" for you.**

- **Never take family for granted. Their love and support is unconditional.**

- **Enjoy the journey. It is not a destination.**

CHAPTER EIGHT

Life is a Series of Useful Lessons

by Patricia A. Gabow, MD

As I am about to announce my retirement, the invitation to update the original 1995 monograph has provided an opportunity to reflect on all the events and attitudes that have helped shape my entire career. In this reflection, I have come to realize that there are no major differences in the guiding principles of my personal and professional lives. In the next several pages, I will try to pass on the advice I have derived from many good and wise people over the years and share the lessons they have taught.

Because these lessons were not read from a book, the first step to success is to seek friends and mentors from whom you can learn at every point in your life—nothing else will serve you so well both as a person and as a professional. I have decided to name the people who helped me as a kind of thank you to each of them. Some of them may think I was not particularly attentive to the lessons while they were being taught, and there is more than a grain of truth in that. Some lessons have "sunk in" slowly. Often, I fail to follow the advice even when I believe it to be true. Nonetheless, having these lessons has been invaluable and it is in that spirit that I share them.

Although we cannot choose our families, we all know that they have an enormous influence on our futures. I was very fortunate to have an exceptional and warm extended family that taught me most of the important lessons for success. My grandparents came to this country from Italy in the early 1900s. Both my grandfathers arrived as adolescents—alone and with nothing. Their experiences taught me not to be afraid to take a risk. My mother reinforced this willingness to accept risk, encouraging me to attend medical school—something virtually unheard of in the rural Italian immigrant community in which I grew up. This reinforcement or restating of a lesson has been a common occurrence; wise people often seem to espouse similar philosophies.

My maternal grandfather was a wonderfully wise, peasant philosopher with insights into all aspects of life. He had an array of old sayings that are worth understanding. Let me share one that greatly influenced me from childhood through this day: "If you have a gift and you don't use it, no confessor on earth can absolve you." Hearing this repeatedly ingrained in me the concept that any talents a person has are "given" with the obligation to use them in service. More than thirty years later, Dr. Samuel Their, another mentor, taught the same lesson. He believed that medicine was a learned profession in which practitioners are given valued information from the previous generation that we are to use, enrich, and pass on to the next generation without undue rewards. Lesson: Use your talents in service.

Both my parents taught me that natural gifts and talents require hard work to be brought to fruition. In my school days, this was translated into "If you have the ability to get an A by working very hard, a B with minimal work is not acceptable." Lesson: Always do your absolute best.

My mother taught me another valuable lesson while I was in grade school. My school was in a rural area of Pennsylvania, and many children in my class were so poor, they often came day after day in the same dirty clothes. My mother, who was a school teacher, reached out to everyone, especially these children, putting into action what she told me, "Be nice to everyone, especially the poor children." Lesson: Reach out to everyone.

I see many people in leadership positions, especially physicians and academicians, who see themselves as above the crowd and deserving of different treatment than housekeepers, food service people, clerks, etc. This class mentality does not serve a leader well. I might add that this lesson, stated in work and deed so many times over many years, may be the single most important reason why I have spent my entire academic career in a city/county hospital.

Still another lesson came from the older generation of women in my extended Italian family. By today's standards, they had tough lives. They had very large families; they did all the work themselves—the cooking, cleaning, washing, canning—on and on. I can't remember my paternal grandmother ever going on vacation or ever being taken out to dinner. My father was killed in World War II, and it was many years before my mother remarried. None of these women ever complained or were morose or bitter. In fact, they had great joy for life.

Lesson: Don't whine—look at the good things in your situation. My grandfather had an old saying for this as well: "Not everything bad happens to harm you."

Sister Florence Marie Scott was my mentor during my four college years. The college was a Catholic girls' school where, at least in those days, every class started with a prayer chosen by the teacher. Head of the biology department, Sister Florence, began every class with the same prayer, which ended, "...grant that I may understand the truth, and, when I understand the truth, fire me with the courage to use it." As you enter leadership positions, you will confront difficult problems. In these instances, it is critical to try your best to understand the truth and not just accept what you'd like to hear. Leadership positions at any level tend to be addictive; you like the role. It becomes difficult to be willing to put the job (or for that matter, advancement to the next job) on the line by defending with vigor and zeal a position that you see as true, but is unpopular. In some sense, I have come to believe people who have leadership positions should be those who don't want to keep them at any cost. They must feel free to make the right decisions even if it could cost them their jobs.

Sister Florence also reinforced the concept of risk taking. In those days, when nuns wore habits and were largely confined to convents, Sister was on the board of directors of the Marine Biological Laboratories in Woods Hole (the first and only woman at the time—let alone the only nun!). She spent every summer doing her research there. In this environment, she remained a nun— right down to wading in the water to collect specimens with her habit tucked around her legs. This sent a very loud and clear message—a woman can succeed in a man's world without changing who or what she is.

Medical school and housestaff training brought many mentors and lessons and much advice, but I will focus on two special mentors. Dr. Samuel Their, head of the housestaff program and Dr. Arnold Relman, as chief of medicine gave the same, very clear message—set high standards for people you supervise and they will work to meet those standards. In a leadership role, clearly stating the standards and goals sets the tone for everyone in an institution and by setting them, you give people your support to be stars.

I clearly remember another lesson taught by Dr. Relman. One day, making rounds, he said, "There are many forces conspiring to kill the patient; the doctor should not be one of them." Of course, no one was actually trying to kill the patient. The reference was to giving the best care. In a time when marketplace forces may not always be aimed at the best interests of the patient, this lesson must especially be embraced by physician executives. They have a professional obligation not shared by other executives.

The corollary to Dr. Relman's lesson was to be the best physician you can be. From my perspective, being a good doctor may be the best possible training for being a health care executive—the operating principles are the same. To solve a problem, as in treating a patient, you need to make a diagnosis, develop a treatment plan, implement it, monitor the outcome, and change the treatment and/or rethink the diagnosis if you're not getting the response you expect. Sometimes, in both medicine and administration, you have to start out by treating a symptom, but you shouldn't be fooled into thinking that the symptom is the disease. When I was Chief of Medicine, I used to tell the housestaff that it only took a few things to be a great house officer: listening to the patient, caring about the patient, being compulsive about getting the needed data, and being able to pick up the phone and ask for help when you need it. The same applies to being a good administrator, except instead of the patient, you need to listen to the people in the institution and care about its well-being.

When I started my working life at Denver Health and Hospitals and the University of Colorado School of Medicine, I was fortunate to have mentors who remain my advisors to this day. From Dr. Schrier at the University, I learned to "hang in there." An example of this was his efforts to get a cigarette tax on the state's ballot to help pay for health care for the poor. He worked tirelessly on this for eight years Every failed attempt was responded to with a new strategy and finally Colorado did get a cigarette tax which has provided many millions of dollars to health care in the state. So the lesson is, if something is important to do, keep trying until you achieve it. In leading large, complex institutions, this is critical, because they change very slowly and with great difficulty. Persistence and long vision are necessary for success.

Watching Dr. Schrier recruit over many years, I learned another important lesson: surround yourself with the smartest and best people you can. Often, people in leadership positions are threatened by those who may be smarter or more talented than they are. This is a mistake. Having the best people on your team only makes you and your team better.

Another lesson was about pushing yourself. Many times during the early days of my academic career, when I didn't want to try something new, such as giving grand rounds or starting a research lab, I'd hear the message, "If you don't stretch, you won't grow."

The last lesson I learned from Dr. Schrier was about praising people. This goes beyond the pat on the back and the thank you note. Let me give you one example. When I was promoted to associate professor, Dr. Schrier wrote my parents a letter! My mother has never forgotten that. Personal caring like this creates a loyalty and esprit de corps on a team that is hard to beat. (Parenthetically, this is a recurrence of my mother's message about reaching out.)

Dr. Sbarbaro, my mentor at Denver Health and Hospitals, taught me two lessons when I first became Chief of Medicine: only touch the same piece of paper once and don't be afraid to make decisions. He went on to say that if you never make a decision, you'll never make a good one. On the other hand, if you aren't afraid to make decisions, at least some of them will be right. To succeed in this fast-paced life, you need to make as many decisions as are feasible on round one, move on, and don't agonize later. If the decision is wrong, learn from it, but don't wring your hands over it. This principle is another one that has strong grounding in the practice of medicine and its teaching tool, the mortality and morbidity (M&M) conference. As Chief of Medicine, I always told the housestaff that they must expect to make some mistakes, but they must also try not to make the same mistake twice. The M&M conference teaches that it is healthy to put those mistakes on the table and discuss them. We, in fact, have done some administrative M&M conferences, and I think physician administrators should use this tool more often.

Dr. Sbarbaro taught me another important lesson. You can have a knockdown, drag out disagreement about an issue with someone, walk away, and not be mad—disagreeing about a matter is not a personal attack by you or on you.

I'd like to end with what I have learned from my husband and children. One cannot be guaranteed a wonderful spouse, but I have had this blessing. I cannot personally overestimate the professional accomplishments that have been made possible by having a stable and happy marriage. Many people move from one institution to another as a means of advancing their careers. Although I am certain that is a valid approach, being at one institution for an entire career is not unlike having one husband—you really get to know and care about the institution in a very special way. For me, having started as an entry level physician straight out of fellowship and moving through the system has been invaluable. You know the system from the bottom up, with all its strengths and quirks. Even more important, you know the people in the institution and in the community.

My husband, Hal, has also taught me that, when you're uncertain about something, always assume the best. This especially applies to people. If you are fortunate enough to have children, they will teach more valuable lessons about administration than probably any other teachers—such great truths as don't nag, don't take yourself too seriously, don't sweat the small stuff, don't play favorites, one "bad" action doesn't mean someone is a "bad" person, put some sugar in the medicine, and give lots of hugs and kisses (figuratively, of course).

Finally, the admonition I like best of all is "get a life"—which I think means, see the big picture or get out of your little world. Or maybe it doesn't mean that. This, of course, is a critical point; you have to learn to live comfortably with ambiguity.

In addition to this long litany of what I have been taught by others, I actually think I learned one thing on my own (although, if I think about it for a while, probably someone taught it to me too.). As I moved in my career from head of the renal division to Chief of Medicine to Deputy Manager to Chief Executive Officer of Denver Health and Hospitals, it has become apparent that my vision had to change for each new level of position. The higher you move in an organization, the broader your vision must become and the longer view into the future you must take. This is, in fact, the thrill of leadership.

In 2012, I find that the opportunity to continue to reflect on my career and its lessons is very timely. In 1995 when I first wrote about my transition from clinician to medical manager, I was at the beginning of my leadership career. Now I am approaching its formal ending, having recently announced my plans to retire as Denver Health's CEO at the end of August 2012.

When I retire, I will have been at Denver Health for almost forty years, will have been CEO for twenty years, and will see age seventy in my not too distant future. With these years of added perspective, I still affirm all of the leadership lessons I wrote about in 1995. I have lived them and used them over almost four decades and they have stood the test of time. I will underscore four of them. There are many lessons to be learned from wise people—some family and some strangers, some younger and some older, and some physicians and some politicians.

1) No matter your age or your experience, never stop listening to those who can teach and inspire.

2) If you have some success as a leader and have an opportunity to provide influence, try to understand the truth and have the courage to say what must be said.

3) Remember the words of one of my mentors, Dr. Relman, "As physician executives we are here first and foremost for the patients, not to enrich ourselves or our organizations".

4) My Grandfather always reminded me that patience is a virtue—it is also a necessity for leaders. Few, if any meaningful accomplishments happen quickly. Transitioning Denver Health from a department of city government to an independent entity was more than a five year journey with twists and turns. The effort was transformational; stopping at some turn would have cost Denver Health its future. Embedding Toyota Production Systems or Lean into Denver Health and reaping the benefits was a multiyear journey. Yet, it too has been transformational and stopping at some barrier would also have cost Denver Health's its future. Over time, as efforts reach fruition, the barriers seem to fade from one's memory and only the accomplishment stays vivid (I suspect this is a particular quirk of the lens of time. Let's continue to take on the hard tasks and see them through to the end).

While these lessons from my early years remain guideposts, the years have also added new ones that relate directly to leading a large and complex organization. One of the main obligations of a leader is to create a vision for the organization—a vision which inspires—a vision which is good and noble—a vision which imparts to all employees the belief that they can do great things. Our vision at Denver Health is to be a model for the nation—both audacious and good at a time when our country is sorely in need of models. The vision must be transformed into a path of actions that the leader and those she/he leads can walk. Leaders of large enterprises have many fires to put out every day. Without a path to walk to a greater end, it is easy to feel frustrated and beleaguered. It is this advancement—no matter how small—along the path to achieve vision that gives the work joy. Leaders, like parents, must walk the path they espouse. They must be role models in their professional and personal lives; they must do what they want and expect of others and avoid doing what they do not want others to do. Leaders must commit to organizational transparency and openness. Information is power and it needs to be shared.

Here, in 2012, I think the hardest lesson for a leader must be knowing when to leave. I cannot say I learned it; I can only say I made that decision. But I know deciding to leave my leadership position and Denver Health has pulled at my heart strings. Perhaps, in the end, truly loving your institution and loving what you do everyday, is what it means to be a leader.

CHAPTER NINE

Be Yourself, Everyone Else is Already Taken.

— *Oscar Wilde*

by Jayne McCormick, BSN, MD, MBA

PERSONAL BARRIERS

"There are no constraints on the human mind, no walls around the human spirit, no barriers to our progress except those we ourselves erect."

— *Ronald Reagan*

I've always wanted to be a doctor. When I was young, I always watched the doctor shows on TV. I loved Chad Everett on Medical Center! My personal barrier: I hated school. A recurring challenge of mine, as I have come to realize: I get bored easily and as the expression goes I don't "suffer fools gladly".

My parents wanted me to have a good Catholic education. I hated it. A bunch of well-meaning women, who were never trained to teach, had poor relationship skills and provided poor role models. No intellectual stimulation. My first challenge—and lesson—fight for what you want. Don't be complacent, especially about your education. I campaigned one whole summer and talked my parents into letting me go to public junior high. I was the first in my family to do this. That was my first big achievement.

Public school was better. By 12th grade I was bored again, so I talked myself into becoming a nurse even though I really wanted to be a doctor. I figured 4 more years was all I could stand. So initially, I was erecting my own barriers. Some of us like to do things the hard (and long) way. I'm certainly one of those people. So instead of taking 8 years to get to the end of medical school, it eventually took me 13.

Mabel was my first role model. Mabel was my grandmother and about the only medical person in my family. Business careers are big in my family. She was a nurse in 1910 during a time when very few women had careers. One memorial day, as we visited my grandfather's grave, she told me she had been tending that grave for over 50 years. I had a huge AHA moment—she had been a widow longer than she had been married. The fact that she had a career during an era when most women were housewives, allowed her to remain independent, have a successful career and provide for her family. It made me realize that I should never depend on anyone else to provide for me. I had to be self reliant and find a reliable career for myself. She was an incredibly strong, admirable woman. She was the one everyone looked up to and called if they were ill or had a problem. Mabel persevered till age 95. She was a huge influence on me.

BARRIER: LACK OF ROLE MODELS AND CHALLENGES

"The strongest principle of growth lies in human choice."

— George Eliot

Looking back now, I don't regret taking the longer path through nursing. It was a great 5 years. The experience has given me a nursing perspective that as a health care leader I now find invaluable. Nurses are our frontline and I have walked in their shoes. Initially, I loved the medicine and taking care of patients. I worked in a burn unit and fell in love with the multidisciplinary team approach. Surgical residents rotated through the unit. They made the major decisions about patient care. I realized that I wanted to have more influence on my patient's care. It was a critical care unit and we also staffed our own operating room. I fell in love with the comradery of the OR and the excitement of critical care. After a year or two, I realized nursing wasn't satisfying enough for me. Even though I had already started my masters in nursing, I wanted to be more involved with creating treatment plans and making decisions. I also felt a void—no mentors that I could relate to in nursing. While riding on a ski lift one day, a surgery resident unknowingly made a huge impact on my life. He advised me against going to medical school and on to a surgical residency. He told me the work would be too hard. His implication—a woman wouldn't make it. The gauntlet was thrown down! Challenge accepted, decision made.

BARRIERS: TIME AND STEREOTYPES

AGE IS NO BARRIER

"Don't presume to tell me what I will and will not do. You don't know me".

— Titanic

Another hurdle—I had to go back to school before I could even apply to medical school. You would think that nursing school would have been great preparation. Unfortunately I had to go back and get Physics, Calculus, Organic Chemistry and more English. I decided, if I did well and persevered it would be an omen that I should go on to medical school. So while my friends were all getting married and starting families, I went back to undergraduate school. About that time I realized I was becoming pretty driven.

I remember a discussion earlier with some of my high school girlfriends—they all had these big career plans. They were shocked that I wouldn't consider marrying a manager of McDonald's. They thought I was a snob. I wasn't. I just didn't realize yet that if I married, I wanted someone who would respect me and whom I would totally respect. A good career was extremely important to me and I wanted my husband to have a strong one as well. I wanted us to be equals. Again, self reliance is an important value for me and has been part of my success. Interestingly enough, none of those friends focus on their careers now. They have chosen to focus on family. I believed then, as now, that you can have both and be satisfied with both.

> "I don't believe you have to be better than everybody else. I believe you have to be better than you ever thought you could be."
>
> *— Ken Venturi*

It was difficult to pick up and leave my friends and go back to school full time. However, I loved the intellectual challenge of medical school. Dating however was tough. The guys were pretty intimidated that I wanted to be a surgeon. My ambition didn't go too well with their egos. Plus, the other students thought I was so old. I was a whole five years older. No women role models in medical school that I remember even though it was the late 1980's and 40 percent of my class was female. In fact my surgery chairman told me that women shouldn't go into surgery. Oh my God! It was like waving a red cape in front of me again! No way would I back down now. Would you believe that when I went to interview for residency positions, one of the male physician interviewers asked me if I had ever sewn clothes growing up? As if this was a qualification? I wanted to ask him how much he had done in high school. Needless to say I didn't rank that place.

I ended up going to Eastern Virginia Graduate School of Medicine for my surgical residency. I tried to interview at the other two surgical residencies in Virginia but at that time they rarely considered women. At Eastern Virginia, I finally found some mentors. There were no female professors or attendings when I first started, but there were several female senior residents (one per year). One of my chiefs was a woman. Finally someone I could look up too. Also on faculty was a black male trauma surgeon which was quite amazing considering this was the south. He was one of the best teachers I ever had, a real mover and shaker. He kept you on your toes. He told me no female had ever made it through their trauma rotation as a chief without calling in sick. In other words women were weak. So what did I do? I volunteered to take the hardest rotation that year. We were short a resident, so I worked consecutive 36 hour rotations for over a month and never missed a day. No 80 hour work weeks then. I have a habit of proving things (and competing with) myself. It was also an unwritten rule that surgery residents didn't miss any time for childbearing. So being a fool, I timed it so my first child would be born just after I finished. Pregnancy as a chief surgical resident was no fun! Oops! My water broke 3 weeks early, in the OR during a Thoracotomy. Of course I finished the case and finished the year.

ASSET: WORK LIFE BALANCE

"If you obey all of the rules, you miss all of the fun"

— *Katherine Hepburn*

I married during my residency. I swore I would never marry another physician. And I didn't want children. I didn't want interference with my career. So, who do I marry? I ended up marrying a "fertility" doctor. Fate was laughing at me! The best laid plans... My husband has not been any barrier. I met him as an intern, he understands my world. He has always known how important my career is to me and has never questioned or been threatened by it. He is always supportive and very willing to share. He has taken on child rearing responsibilities when needed. He's not stuck in traditional marriage roles. We share many of the same interests. I love the outdoors, physical fitness and animals. Work life balance is so important. I have been able to achieve that. I do work very hard. But as they say, I play hard. Mucking out stalls, breaking horses, holding onto a hormonally crazed stallion during breeding season, and hiking in the Sandia Mountains helps me maintain balance. What I initially thought would be a barrier has become very important to my "success". It has also reminded me to be flexible and to change with life's circumstances.

RIGHT PLACE AT THE RIGHT TIME

FINALLY SOME MORE MENTORS!

"You must be the change you wish to see in the world"

— Mahatma Gandhi

My first year as a "real" surgeon was in academics in Virginia. Research and teaching aren't my strength, although I loved working with the residents. They keep you mentally sharp. I helped cover the trauma service which initially was exciting, but the thrill was soon gone. That year allowed me to learn the academic view of medicine which I have also found very helpful in my health care career. I often find my hospital systems competing with academic medical centers. It helps to understand "where they are coming from".

However, at that point, I liked building longer term relationships with patients. After my husband completed his fellowship, I moved on to private practice in Nebraska. While there, I started getting involved in elected medical staff positions. As they say, I became an "accidental" leader. (I kept making the mistake of saying yes). I loved it. I had two female chiefs of staff in particular who influenced me. An eclectic psychiatrist and a down to earth, do the right thing kind of radiologist. They both encouraged me to get involved in physician leadership. I started seeing the bigger picture in health care. I realized there is more to medicine than taking care of patients, one at a time. I started to embrace the vision of physicians as a key group needed to create affordable, quality, health care.

Clinically, however, I started to get bored again. After my thousandth cholecystectomy, I was wondering what's next. Around that time, I helped care for several cancer patients, none of whom had experienced what I considered a "good death". I learned about Hospice. I started educating myself about the new specialty of Hospice and Palliative Care medicine. People can have a good death and actually live longer if we focus on quality of life and not quantity of life. I realized there was a huge need for End of Life Care in our society. Many people are unaware of the benefits of Hospice and Palliative care. I started gaining a non-surgical perspective in health care. Ironically at about that time, the medical director of my affiliated organization's Hospice died (from cancer). I became the Hospice medical director. This move had a huge impact on me. It was one of my first "paid" management/leadership positions and has truly added an important, "medical" viewpoint to my leadership portfolio. I loved it so much that after several years, I decided to leave surgery. The new field called to me. I become a Palliative Care doctor. I am now double boarded in Surgery and Hospice and Palliative Care Medicine.

OPPORTUNITY: RIGHT PLACE AT RIGHT TIME

BARRIER: MISPERCEPTIONS

My darling girl, when are you going to understand that "normal" isn't a virtue? It rather denotes a lack of courage."

— *Practical Magic*

Fate again stepped in. My organization hired a new CMO. He was one of the most strategic people I have ever met! He preached a new vision of health care. He understood the importance of paid, physician leadership. He was willing to invest time and money in physician leaders. He had a new idea for quality officers at each of our metropolitan hospitals. I was the first woman he asked to become one. New challenge? Different path? Of course I would take it. My surgical partner thought I had lost my mind. How could I "throw away" all those years of training in surgery? My other colleagues thought I had gone to "the dark side" and wasn't a real doctor any more. It blows my mind how many doctors think that just because you are paid by a hospital or health system that all free thought has flown out of you head! Huge barrier, but I have learned that with time, through relationship building and the development of trust, those misperceptions can be overcome.

Around that time a chief quality officer for the system was also hired. Now we had two strong physician leaders. Both were men and both had a huge impact on me. The CQO was a great mentor who was actually looking out for my interests. He was interested in "growing me" as a leader. A rare opportunity arose. I was in the right place at the right time. The CMO was developing a physician executive leadership/MBA program with Gallup University and the University of Nebraska. I was asked to take part in the pilot group. There were only nine of us in that class, all physicians. Working full time, raising two teenagers and going to school for an MBA was going to be very difficult, but I figured this opportunity might not present itself again.

One of the best things I ever did. I grew so much! The first unit in the course was "knowing self". I believe that to be a good leader you really have to take a good look at yourself, warts and all. That program allowed me to be very introspective. We did an analysis that involved the "strengths finder" program. My first strength is "responsibility". This is a huge part of why I am so obsessive about getting things done. The course teaches you that a strength, if not controlled, can turn into a barrier. I'm also an "achiever"—I always have to move onto the next challenge. As a "learner", I need "input" which is why I constantly require so much data. I am also strong in "harmony" which I think is one of the most important things I have learned to utilize. If you don't take the time to build relationships, forget it. Not a lot of physicians have this strength and I have seen this deficit adversely affect my mentors.

The third unit in the leadership portion of the course was learning the global perspective. This portion was so important and eye opening. We traveled to Thailand and looked at medical tourism. One beautiful facility (Bumrungrad Hospital) was Joint Commission certified, had staff with a great service orientation and provided high quality care at a much cheaper price than the U.S. Huge AHA! We Americans incorrectly always assume our health care is better!

LESSON LEARNED: SERVANT LEADER

OPPORTUNITIES EVEN IN ADVERSITY

"A woman is like a tea bag; you never know how strong it is until it's in hot water."

— *Eleanor Roosevelt*

I completed my MBA in 2009. My children were so proud of their graduate. Shortly after, my professional world imploded. My mentors, in their attempt to improve quality and move the organization forward, I feel, forgot to build relationships and listen. I read a recent article on the negative aspects of silence in the work place. To this day, I feel I should have been more vocal and courageous. I started to see that my leaders were heading down the wrong path and I think "what if" I had been more vocal in trying to get them to stop and build more relationships. These two physicians had such vision, but without relationship skills and the ability to listen to others, they sank. A big upheaval occurred. The medical staff voted no confidence in the administration. The CEO, VP, CMO and several others all "resigned". The organization became so afraid of physician leadership that, in my opinion, they have taken "two steps backward".

This was a huge learning experience for me! With time, despite the personal and professional setback, I was able to learn and grow from this tough experience. My realization—I wanted to continue to be a physician leader. Collaborate, listen, change course when you are wrong; trust and relationship building is what it is all about. Unfortunately, to continue to grow professionally, I realized I would have to move elsewhere.

HUGE PERSONAL BARRIER: IT'S ALL ABOUT WHO YOU KNOW

"Life is a banquet and most poor suckers are starving to death"

— *Auntie Mame*

For a woman to pick up and leave for a new job opportunity, I feel, is a lot harder than for a man. I had several barriers. My daughter had one more year in High School. She is valedictorian and a cross country star. Could I ask her to leave that? My husband was willing to stay, bless him. Even my closest friends and family couldn't believe I would "leave" my family. People constantly ask my poor son how he is doing without his mother. Military men leave all the time. They don't get all these questions. It was and continues to be extremely difficult to live apart from my family who are my support system. However I felt strongly that this opportunity came at the right time. Or maybe not exactly the right time, but when a great opportunity arises, I feel you have to grab it or be left behind. A colleague I had befriended while I was earning my MBA called about a position in New Mexico. I've learned that networking with colleagues and staying in touch is critical for career advancement. This was the opportunity to become CMO for three metropolitan hospitals in an eight hospital system. It was an opportunity for career growth and probable advancement in the future. It was also in a location that called to my outdoor nature (I knew that kind of opportunity wouldn't come along very often). I interviewed twice and was turned down because they were rethinking the position. I was devastated. I felt I was perfect for the role. After a few months rather than giving up, I began looking at other opportunities. Several months later, New Mexico called me back. They had decided that the original job was too big for one person, instead, dividing it into two jobs. I was asked to return to interview for the metropolitan CMO position. This experience underscores the importance of not burning bridges, even when you are disappointed.

I love my job. I have grown so much since starting. People seem to really invite physician input and leadership here. It has also strengthened and forced me to improve my own mentoring skills. I have concentrated on relationship building and trust development. I am respected and now realize how important this personal value is to me. Although I had it in Nebraska, it was more grudgingly given there. Now, I am concentrating on earning everyone's trust and providing value to my colleagues and our patients. The job isn't easy, but it is challenging.

I have a female mentor again! My boss (the other part of the original job) for the first time in leadership is a woman. Initially, I was worried. She was hired just before me, so I had not gotten a chance to meet her. What a relief when we finally met. She has a great sense of humor, is all about relationships and is very strategic. We are so different. That is another thing I have learned along my career journey. I want to partner with people who are and see things differently. That way we can utilize our strengths to complement each other. You want contrasting and occasionally conflicting view points. I don't ever want tunnel vision. As an old professor taught me, I want to see things from the balcony, not the orchestra. There are many challenges on my horizon. Healthcare is at such an exciting crossroad and I am well positioned to take part. Can't wait for the next challenge!

Thinking back:

My greatest barriers:

- Personal barriers

- Misperceptions

- Sexual stereotypes

- Lack of strong role models

My greatest assets:

- Strong, independent personality

- Continuous need for intellectual challenge

- Took advantage of being in the right place at the right time

- Diverse medical background/perspective

- Mentoring

- Ability to adapt and change

- Work/life balance

"Do not go where the path may lead, go instead where there is no path and leave a trail."

— *Ralph Waldo Emerson*

So, I understand my inner drive now that makes me take roads that are less well traveled. I have also been independent and it is all about personal achievement and not competitiveness, unless it is with me. I am a much different person today from who I was when I started the healthcare journey. I'm glad I took the long route. I'm glad I've had adversity and disappointments. I am stronger for them. Being a woman fighting preconceptions, misperceptions and prejudice has made me tougher than many I know. Leadership has allowed me to come to know myself better than I thought I ever could. I have become so much more intentional about forming relationships and trust. I no longer think about mistakes and defeat, but about opportunities for change and improvement. I love being able to affect a larger group of patients and people in contrast to my days when I operated on one patient at a time. Don't we all just want to know we have made a difference in the world? I know I have and I feel I am just getting started!

CHAPTER TEN

The Journey and the Legacy

by Hoda A. Asmar, MD, MBA, FACPE, FACHE, FACP

I grew up in Beirut, Lebanon, the second of three children and the only girl. Both my parents were illiterate. Because each was working by age ten to support their respective families, they never had an opportunity for an education. War waged in my country all through my middle, high school and medical education. That war experience transformed routine challenges of a simple life into a constant fight against so many odds: weeks and months of interrupted studies, no electricity, no running water, bread lines, geographic confinement, constant sounds of bombs and bullets, vivid images of casualties and atrocities, and the misery of the displaced.

Studying by candlelight for days on end was not fiction and figuring out how to get to the hospital during fuel shortages and under constant bomb shelling was part of attending medical school. Everyone carried arms in those days—from revolvers to M16s and everyone was on edge. Working an emergency department shift was one of the most dangerous places for a medical student or doctor who might be shot by an unhappy patient or family member.

My journey from clinician to medical management began in 1982 with the start of medical school. Despite all the obstacles, the many wonderful expected and unexpected turns along the way have all led to the best career I would have ever hoped for, many happy memories of colleagues, friends and patients and a great sense of satisfaction.

I remember being told that a four years college degree was fine, that I shouldn't strive for anything more. Certainly not medicine. Why would I want to pursue all these years of training, the long hours, the hostile environment of medical school in the Middle East, and the constant struggles to balance work and life? Better to find a nine to five job and maybe my children would become physicians.

Obviously I didn't listen. I graduated from medical school in 1989 and started post-graduate training in Paris, France since I spoke French. There I soon realized that the environment was not a good fit for my aspirations. In 1992, I moved to the US with just three days to sharpen my marginal English skills before scheduled internship interviews for an internal medicine position.

I completed my internal medicine residency at Polyclinic Medical Center, in Harrisburg, Pennsylvania, and my infectious disease fellowship at Hahnemann University Hospital in Philadelphia. I enjoyed my training, and have great memories of superb and supporting faculty, attendings, and peers at both organizations.

In 1998, I started in my first clinical practice in Cadillac, Michigan anticipating a permanent career in direct patient care. At that time I never considered medical management.

Moving from direct patient care to a physician executive role happened more by circumstance than planning. I was in practice in a small rural community and was offered an interim role as a medical director for a ten county public health department in Northern Michigan. As the first infectious disease specialist in the community, I also filled in various leadership roles at the local hospital including managing infection control, employee health, and the newly established hospitalist program.

About a year into clinical practice and my role as medical director in public health, I started a weekend MBA program at Michigan State University. I chose a non-healthcare oriented program, since I was not specifically focused on a full-time physician executive role. At that time I had no specific plan. I just went with the flow, still contemplating a direct patient care career.

In 2000, I took on my first role as part-time Vice President of Medical Affairs at Mercy Hospital in Cadillac where I practiced. This VPMA position seemed a natural expansion of my clinical role as it meant involvement in the medical staff and in the community through public health.

In 2004, I had my son Alex. Suddenly I was faced with the question of how to balance family and work life, how to consider my son's needs and still be able to learn and build my career. Work-life balance has become a continuous refinement process. With the arrival of my son, I made a conscious decision to pursue a full-time career as a physician executive. I moved to a larger 390+ bed hospital within the same Trinity Healthcare system—St. Joseph's Medical Center in Macomb, Michigan. Later on, I was recruited to a large independent hospital in Naperville, Illinois—Edward Hospital & Health Services—where I remained until 2011. At Edward hospital, I created and realigned the hospitalist group, case management and social work departments, and successfully brought an outsourced pharmacy department internally. In addition, I managed many other departments, including clinical excellence, medical records and the Neurosciences Institute.

I am presently the Sr. Vice President, Chief Medical Officer for Presbyterian Healthcare Services in Albuquerque, New Mexico, a highly integrated healthcare system with eight hospitals and the state's largest health plan and multi-specialty employed physician and mid-level providers group.

In each of my successive roles, I added new responsibilities, expanded beyond the traditional role of a chief medical officer and successfully managed operational areas. I am proud of each of these organizations, their teams and my association with them.

At a personal level, I make a point of carving out time to enjoy family, vacations, and long-lasting friendships. I especially love being involved in my son's activities and studies. All of this helps me to reenergize and stay healthy. Part of my approach to balancing work-life, is having a clear vision of goals, an organized approach to tasks and projects, surrounding myself with great teams of subject matter experts, knowing when to delegate, being practical, and realistically assessing time needs for various business and personal tasks. Finally, knowing when to say no, and avoiding personal and work related over-commitment helps.

I am asked on many occasions: "do you miss clinical practice?" and it is always difficult to answer because I don't feel I have moved away from clinical practice as much as I have chosen a "new sub-specialty". I have never wavered from medicine as a career choice.

In my twelve years as a physician executive I learned the importance of the following:

#1 Self-awareness: Before deciding on a journey or career choice, be transparent with yourself about why you are making that choice. What are your expectations? Are you running from something or purposefully going somewhere?

What brings you true satisfaction? Are you just looking for "greener pastures" or do you have a realistic picture of what is ahead?

Understand your own learning and work style, how you interact with others, how you are perceived by others, your sense of values, and what anchors you. Ask yourself these hard questions and seek open and honest feedback from people around you.

#2 Build on past experiences, personal and professional: Dissecting past experiences will help you learn and apply valuable lessons. It will help you decide on career paths, what environment you will thrive in, what type of management style you would relate to, and the important skill of learning to transform a negative experience into a learning step instead of a grudge or regret. The classic "never burn bridges" is always true.

#3 Connect to others: Connect with the people you work with and report to as well as those who report to you and those you meet on interviews, in meetings and in various functions. These experiences are all part of the journey. Be genuine and authentic, observe and learn, and connect more than network.

#4 Build a circle of mentors: Mentors can be other executives (physicians or not), friends, a coach, family members, each in a different way. But the most impactful mentors are the ones who will tell you what you don't want to hear. It is very important that your circle not include just physician executives. You need to communicate and interact with people who come from diverse backgrounds, education and training.

#5 Be inclusive of others: Think the "we" versus "I", believe it and reflect it sincerely. A major skill for physician executives is the ability to function in a team even when you are not the leader, to navigate organizational politics, and to understand the importance of winning together.

#6 Solid accomplishments: Establish a track record of tangible experiences and accomplishments. The ability to "talk the talk" without an objective measurable track record will not last long, especially in this present rapidly changing healthcare environment.

#7 Take risks: The most reward comes from a big challenge, so learn to take and manage risks. Expect some failures. This is not a career for the highly risk averse or the physician who prefers a strict, well-defined career path. Again, you have to be self-aware to know how much risk you can handle and why and when to take it.

#8 Build a reputation of honesty, and integrity: In a professional circle where unfortunately not everyone has a reputation for being honest with peers, mentors, and colleagues, someone with a strong sense of values and integrity is priceless. It is also important to show gratitude toward those who help and support you along the way.

#9 Share knowledge: Be a team player, build consensus and share power. Hoarding information and knowledge will reduce your influence. Encourage and practice transparency within your team, reports and organization. Being a role model and mentoring others is part of knowledge sharing too.

 # 10 Focus on the patient: In my day to day work as a CMO and when I am facing a challenge, or a difficult decision, I always return to my original clinical focus point and consider "what is in the best interest of our patients?"

#11 Career moves: Some may advise never to make a lateral move, but that is not always possible. Any position change should be well thought out, be it part of a growth opportunity, a long-term strategy, a clear move up, getting out of a bad fit situation, or stepping into something that gives you more personal satisfaction.

#12 Be a constant learner: Never stop learning, reading, observing, and trying new ways. Challenge yourself: What can I improve? How can I grow? Be insightful about your own abilities and shortcomings, and focus on your personal continued improvement.

#13 Understand your organizational culture: An executive needs to appreciate organizational politics, know how to add value, ask pertinent questions, and have a good grasp of the organizational culture. Ignoring that aspect of your role will limit your success and ability to have a strong impact.

In the end, making career choices is highly individual. Each person should go through a self-assessment to discern what brings them satisfaction and success. I see myself as continuously pursuing roles that make a difference, and are impactful. In my opinion, the future is all about the people you meet along the journey and the legacy you leave behind.

CHAPTER ELEVEN

Medical Manager: Was It Worth It?

by Selma Harrison Calmes, MD

This chapter is about my 20 years as a department chair in anesthesiology in two public (county) hospitals. In many ways, my experience as a female medical manager was unique, but I hope the lessons learned will be useful to others. My management experience was different than most because it focused on anesthesiology and operating rooms (ORs). At the time, the surgeons ruled, and there was little interest at the hospital level on intelligent use of OR time, resources and revenue generation.

I decided to be a physician after having polio at age eight during one of California's many polio epidemics. I was hospitalized for months. The trauma of being hospitalized for polio then is only now being realized as recently published patient memoirs vividly document the psychic trauma and family disruption. Like most polio survivors, I ignored the psychic effect of hospitalization and the residual physical effects of the disease. Super-achievement was also a by-product of polio; most survivors are classic Type A personalities. Although I'd been paralyzed initially, I eventually managed to pass as "normal", in spite of a slight limp. Nevertheless, trying to do so took enormous physical effort.

My family was already stressed before polio. My mother was an "Army brat," whose goal in life was to be a colonel's wife and have beautiful children. My father was the son of a Swedish immigrant steel mill worker. After working in the same steel mill, he joined the Army, was able to go to West Point and launch a successful military career. In 1944, he was killed in action in Germany, leaving my mother a 26-year-old widow with three children under age four. I was the oldest; the youngest was only three months old. In contrast to the many programs to support families of those lost in current wars, in World War II, there were few resources to help families like ours, except for a small monthly payment from Social Security. You were just on your own.

Like most women of the time, my mother was totally unprepared to make a living and raise three children alone. I realize now that she was probably too depressed to give her children the emotional support we needed after the loss of our dad; she was struggling herself. As we grew up, money was always very limited. Academic and athletic achievement was expected as a way out of poverty and to repeat the pattern of our dad's life achievements. Despite the fact that being a smart female was definitely discouraged in the 1950s-60s, I managed to make it through a prestigious college on scholarships by living at home and by taking every possible student job. I was fortunate to get into medical school with the help of my organic chemistry professor.

Although it was physically stressful, I loved medical school and I loved being a doctor. The interactions with patients, especially children and their families, solving the puzzle of what was wrong with the patient as well as the "doing" in surgery and anesthesia were exactly what I wanted. I decided on anesthesia during a pediatric internship, on the advice of the women pediatricians with whom I worked. They felt that anesthesia was a good specialty for a woman with children because the hours were allegedly better than in other specialties. I later found this to be an urban legend!

At that time, most hospitals had moderate surgical schedules, and OR work generally ended in the afternoon. However, cases often ran late or emergencies rolled in and sometimes fellow anesthesia staff got sick. So there were many times when I was up all night on-call. Today, because the OR is usually the only profit center for institutions, ORs are pushed to turn out as many cases as possible as efficiently as possible. ORs now typically have at least two shifts for elective surgery, and all the emergencies then follow. The modern practicing anesthesiologist usually doesn't get dinner until 8:30 PM or later, and then start the emergency cases. Room turn-over time (the time to get the OR cleaned and set up for the next case) is tracked, and care of a patient with an anesthesia problem can be marginalized due to this "production pressure".

My management training began while I was trying to be a wife and mother AND a physician. I'd married a medical school classmate after freshman year, had a baby during internship and then another during residency, so anesthesia's disruptive work hours became difficult. It took a household staff of five (four were part-time) to meet all my family's needs and an accountant to deal with all the workers' paperwork. In desperation, I started reading basic books about management, hoping to manage my life more easily and make room for some fun.

About this time, I also wondered how women physicians in the past had managed their families while practicing medicine. This led to a strong interest in the history of women in medicine, an area that has become an exciting academic endeavor for me. Incidentally, the answer to the question about how past women physicians managed is that they either were unmarried, stopped practice once they married, or had live-in servants.

My first job in anesthesia was at a children's hospital in central California where I was one of three anesthesiologists. After seven years, I'd done everything you could do in pediatric anesthesia at the time, so I looked for a new opportunity. Opting for academics, I took a part-time job as the first pediatric anesthesiologist at a university hospital in Los Angeles, about 200 miles away. My success teaching there two days a week ultimately led to a divorce and a move to Los Angeles with two children. In those days, the academic promotion system was secretive, and the importance of research was not made obvious to women who were told that teaching and clinical care were sufficient to excel. Male physicians, on the other hand, seemed to get picked up and mentored by senior colleagues with research labs. After seven years in this position, I learned that my failure to produce research papers meant no promotion.

My next position was as the first specialty anesthesiologist in the state's largest HMO. Daily work assignments were on a strict rotation basis, and I often missed doing the difficult pediatric cases. This was a dysfunctional department filled with many non-performers, including a physician who resented my recent academic experience (I was still on the lecture circuit when I started there). This doctor was an uncontrolled, equal-opportunity and highly experienced bully, my first experience with this problem since medical school. As I studied the day-to-day processes within the department, I recognized areas that needed change and thought about potential solutions. These were my initial insights into how department management might work and the first time I considered a management role for myself.

After failing to make partnership in that organization, I participated in the job fair at our specialty society's annual meeting and quickly received an offer to become chief at a public hospital in central California. Although I hadn't held any prior medical management position, I felt what I had learned while trying to balance medical practice and home life (two children and a husband) would serve as good training for the role.

Like my previous organization, the quality of staff and practice structure was less than optimal, reflecting anesthesiology in that era. The hospital accepted both indigent and private patients. Anesthesia staff were hired by the county at a low basic salary, which was to cover care to the indigent patients. A practice plan existed for private patients who were billed at the usual private fees. That revenue was not shared, but went directly to the anesthesiologist involved. With fierce competition for the private cases, it was hard to find physicians willing to take on county patients. Changing to shared-private practice revenue, common today among anesthesia groups, would mean disrupting the entire practice plan for all the other specialties and was not possible.

One of the most difficult physicians under my supervision was actually mentally ill. He often left his anesthetized patients and wandered in the hallway. At the time, there were no national standards for anesthesia monitoring. Fortunately today there are clear-cut monitoring standards, including continuous presence of the anesthesia providers in the OR. This doctor ended up harassing me for years, making threatening phone calls and breaking into my computer. This was extremely traumatizing.

The medical director who had recruited me was my mentor, the only one I've ever had. He introduced me to the American College of Physician Executives (ACPE). Although he only stayed one year at that hospital, I continued to attend ACPE seminars and read helpful books. There were few anesthesiologists in ACPE then, which would have been useful, because our management problems were and are unique. Anesthesiologists have since formed their own management organization, and many have or are seeking MBAs. We are also taking on leadership roles in the entire perioperative process, preparing patients for surgery and doing postop care, especially in ICUs.

After two years, I moved back to Los Angeles to become chief of anesthesia at another county hospital that was part of a five hospital system. My charge was to get the anesthesiology department affiliated with the associated medical school. That meant recruiting higher quality anesthesia staff –a difficult task given the low salaries.

Much of my administrative time was spent on personnel and budget issues. At one point, the county had an acute budget problem, and I had to lay off half the staff. Union rules required that anesthesiologists from other county institutions be transferred to our hospital, replacing those who were laid-off. All were inadequate clinically, and numerous clinical disasters followed. Trying to deal with this situation was another time-consuming battle, especially because the medical director at the time did not appreciate the need for competent staff.

The surgery faculty was also an issue. They were more interested in doing private cases at their academic hospital, leaving surgery residents in charge of some critically ill indigent patients.

Despite the many obstacles and without a mentor or formal management training, I was slowly able to affect improvements, developing a responsive, communicative, helpful, available department—the only one like that in the hospital at that time. The fact that our group was primarily female might be a good lesson for male medical students and faculty!

Among the positive changes was a medical student rotation that became extremely popular. We also accepted a high-quality CRNA school that had lost its academic home, allowing us better, higher-quality staffing to get the cases done. We initiated a Preoperative Evaluation Clinic staffed by a nurse practitioner we trained. Eventually we took over many aspects of preop patient preparation for surgery including cardiac evaluation. Once I discovered the usefulness of data and the ability to analyze it in Excel, I began keeping basic OR statistics, then added in our Quality Improvement (QI) data. When an OR scheduling system was to be implemented, hospital administration put me in charge, much to the surgeons' chagrin. They never really utilized it; the chair of surgery told me, "I don't believe in data!" I, however, could hardly wait until the end of the month when we could run the statistics to see how we were doing! Although I never received credit for these efforts, I feel validated by the fact that today data management is a vital skill for medical managers.

Meanwhile, in my personal life, polio was rearing its ugly head again. Post-Polio Syndrome (PPS) symptoms (increasing weakness and fatigue in those who had polio[1]) suddenly appeared. There symptoms are aggravated by stress—unavoidable in my position. A major stressor was an unsupportive medical director. Also, anesthesia involves a lot of physical work, and as my symptoms increased, I had to spend less and less time in the OR. Eventually I was forced out of the chair position and into a lateral move to hospital QI. That same week, I discovered a major problem in my marriage. Devastated and totally burnt out, I retired in 2007. After 42 years in medicine, I spent the next two years doing nothing but working in my garden, enjoying its beauty and the natural world.

Now looking back on my career, I wonder whether it was worth trying to be a medical manager. I had a deep personal commitment to public hospitals and indigent care dating from my polio experience when I was a patient in a public hospital. But, I clearly paid a personal price: working in systems chronically stressed by budget problems, aggravation of my PPS, with resultant medical complications, and deterioration of my relationship with my husband. Still, there have been amazing and satisfying rewards: I helped attract many medical students (both male and female) to anesthesia, all of whom saw a department run primarily by women physicians who functioned as a smooth team and gave top patient care. There was no other department like it in the university's environment. This is a gratifying legacy.

The medical director who was my nemesis is gone. My mentee (she was chosen as chair when I left that position) now is the hospital's medical director and discovered the huge mess her predecessor left behind. Some of the medical students who rotated through our department did their anesthesia residencies at our academic hospital and now work as anesthesiologists at that public hospital. Anesthesia residents now rotate through, so the academic affiliation was achieved. And, the patients are still getting great anesthesia care. Policies, such as facilitating breast feeding which I implemented to meet the particular needs of female staff I had hired are still in place. Sexual harassment issues continue to be quickly and effectively dealt with. These are just a few of the reasons for women physicians to consider medical management careers. I believe we bring a unique perspective that can translate into better care for patients, as well as a better work environment for healthcare workers including fellow physicians.

Lessons I learned that might be useful to others include the great importance of data (be the data person in your organization, and understand the information!), look at the big picture (it's easy to miss a good solution if you don't) and use your staff to help generate solutions to management problems. One of the best days for me was after an ACPE program on this. I gathered some staff to discuss a scheduling issue. With only minimum input from me, they came up with an excellent solution! It was so easy, the staff felt empowered and bought into the solution.

Perhaps the hardest lesson I've learned is the importance of communication. You can never communicate too much, in my experience. Although we might think intelligent people who made it through medical school would understand something with one announcement or notice, that is not the case. It takes multiple repeats, in varying ways, to get the message across. I used to get upset with people who missed an announcement/new policy or whatever, but that's just the way it is and we have to keep communicating. Moreover, the staff has to sense your dedication to this. One of the best things I ever did was to post weekly announcements on the main bulletin board. While our hospital was recovering from a major earthquake, I put up announcements every few hours (things were changing rapidly) at the central location where department staff gathered. This turned out to be a critical step to get us functioning as a group after the disaster.

Finally, I want to note that I've found a very satisfying post-retirement work situation as the consultant in anesthesiology for the Los Angeles county coroner's office. I review cases of possible anesthesia-caused deaths and write reports about whether the quality of care was met. This has given me another opportunity to make a difference in anesthesia care; cases with poor management are reported to the state medical board. I also now speak to anesthesia organizations about what I found and how anesthesia care might be improved. The job is much busier than I'd planned, and going to court for hearings and malpractice cases is sometimes unpleasant, but experience in management has helped me handle the multiple aspects of this position, including organizing data and writing well. This has been a wonderful way to "wrap up" a career in medicine. It also seems now like I have a whole new career at an age considered to be elderly!

REFERENCE:

1. Jubelt B, Agre JC. Characteristics and Management of Post-Polio Syndrome. JAMA 2000; 284(4): 412-4

PROVIDER GROUPS

CHAPTER TWELVE

Having Fun While Trying to Have It All

by Josephine Young, MD, MPH

When I was very young, I was often asked what I wanted to be when I grew up. I would reply that I wanted to be a pediatrician and help people. Rather than encouragement, I was advised to consider becoming a nurse or social worker or physician's assistant instead. The message in essence was: with these roles, you can help people, but still have a family life, and not work so hard.

Despite this, with my parents' full support and being driven to follow my heart, I confirmed my decision, in seventh grade, to become a doctor. And now, 33 years after that decision, I am a pediatrician and the Chief Operating Officer of an 80 provider private pediatric group. On the way here, I have been in solo practice, group practice and multi-specialty practice in non-profit, academic and private settings while enjoying a busy and fulfilling life as a wife and mother.

My husband and I both graduated from medical school in 1991, and were married during the week in between our respective medical school graduation ceremonies. After 2 years spent dating from afar, residency as newlyweds felt like another iteration of a long distance relationship. Even with sharing a home, our 3 years of residency were frequently spent apart on-call every third night or more on different nights at different hospitals in different programs. By the time we reached the relative calm of our senior resident year, we decided that it was a good time to start our intended large family. Happily, our oldest was born during my chief resident year.

After residency, I spent just under 2 years in solo practice in a non-profit clinic. While there I also participated as adjunct faculty and resident preceptor. When I resigned, I worked part-time for 3 months in a private pediatrics practice. At the same time, I also served as a continuity clinic attending at the University where I had trained. This short stint was due to the fact that my husband, a newly minted gastroenterologist, had accepted his first faculty job across the country, necessitating a move to Seattle, Washington. Not long after, while pregnant with our second child, I entered a primary care research fellowship. Three years later I had obtained both my MPH and my subspecialty board certification in adolescent medicine. Upon fellowship completion, and while expecting our third child, I returned to private practice in a large multi-specialty non-profit group. I remained there for 2 years before resigning to come to my current practice where I have remained for the past 10 years. During this period we had our fourth child.

As expected, a dual physician marriage imposes significant demands on time and commitment to outside responsibilities. This is especially true as both of us have substantial administrative roles with broad scopes of involvement. While frequently challenging, our profound understanding of each others' professional needs allows us to work with more synergy, less misunderstanding, and more patience. Nevertheless, even with mutual support, intense days are not infrequently encountered.

Looking back over the last 17 years, in spite of having worked in multiple settings, I always anticipated staying long term in each position. However, when organizational priorities undergo substantial change or new opportunities present themselves, it is important not only to be open to options, but also to have the courage to make significant changes. As I adapted and worked in different roles, I have learned important lessons, some more hard won than others. Here are a few I would like to share:

Never go to a meeting to which you do not know the agenda

Corollary: Never attend a meeting to which you do not know the range of attendees.

This lesson was learned early during my chief resident year. Quite unexpectedly one day, my co-chief and I received a phone call from a faculty member requesting our presence at a meeting that afternoon. Not being apprised of the agenda, we naively never thought to ask. Hours later, we walked into a meeting attended by several other faculty members and proceeded to be berated for our handling of a recent housestaff matter. The critique was unwarranted, but being unprepared, we did not have the data at hand for an effective rebuttal.

Since that experience, I always insist on knowing the agenda for any meeting I am asked to attend. As a corollary, I also insist on knowing who will attend the meeting. This serves to minimize surprises or ambushes and also allows me to invite additional attendees to balance the meeting if needed. When built into a habit, these questions about agenda and attendees become very natural to ask at the time of the meeting request. If the gathering is scheduled for a day or more ahead, it is also reasonable to ask for written confirmation including the agenda and list of attendees.

Titles matter

Corollary: **Unless volunteering, ask for compensation before accepting new responsibilities**

When offered my first job out of residency, I was told that while I would be the only doctor on staff, I would not have my predecessor's title of Medical Director because the clinic was in the process of restructuring. Not one to be concerned about titles and organizational hierarchy and not a deliberate negotiator, I was naively ready to agree to the title of staff physician. However, something made me ask how my responsibilities would differ from the previous medical director. Possibly caught off guard, the response was that there would be no difference. Now fully aware of the power play at hand, I suggested that I hold the title of Medical Director until such time as formal changes had been made. Reluctantly, there was agreement.

Two years later, significant management issues came to light that necessitated my direct involvement with the Board of Directors in a confidential meeting. Attempts were made to bar my access to the Board with statements that I had no right of independent access. After a detailed search into the archives, I retrieved the founding Charter and the original organizational chart that defined my right as the Medical Director to have direct access to the Board. Shortly thereafter, I was asked by the Board to assume additional administrative responsibilities, to cover for departed staff including the administrator, and handle all aspects of management, essentially re-building the clinic.

Focused on my dual responsibilities, I waited until the bulk of the urgent work was completed before asking for compensation for these duties. The Board denied my request and told me that I should have asked for this prior to doing the work. This was another hard lesson learned: if I expected compensation for extra work, I needed to make the expectation known and negotiate for it up front rather than waiting for someone else to notice. Several months later, a new administrator was finally hired in replacement. Contingent upon her acceptance of the job were demands that would specifically decrease administrative transparency and accountability. Although this job had a perfect blend of clinical, teaching, and administrative duties for me, I found that the intended organizational structure and oversight was not aligned with my priorities for high quality patient care and institutional integrity. Therefore, I tendered my resignation, giving them 3 months notice to optimize stability for the clinic, and joined the faculty of the university where I had trained.

Throughout this experience, I was fortunate to be mentored by the university's pediatric department chair. As a woman in a prominent leadership position, she gave her time generously, sharing her wisdom and advice. Most importantly, she helped me develop an objective process to examine the situations at hand and determine a course of action that was both prudent and congruent with my management approach. This was the first time that I experienced direct personal mentoring, and she helped me to appreciate the value of asking for and accepting help.

Since then, I have come to fully understand the importance of titles in an organization's hierarchy. It has nothing to do with ego. Rather, a title generally gives the title holder access to information about the organization that he or she would not have without it. Moreover, with a higher title, there is greater access to potential key information that allows for the ability to anticipate and strategize, and to better understand the actions and motivation of other stakeholders in the organization.

As a result of this understanding, I no longer accept new positions without reviewing the organizational chart and knowing where the job title fits. I have also learned to make a conscious decision before taking on new responsibilities as to whether I am investing my time to learn a new skill and whether I need to discuss compensation before I start. This approach has alleviated any sense of unmet expectations.

Define your management philosophy

A writing assignment during my MPH coursework required that I detail my management philosophy. Although many students complained, the professor emphasized that without the ability to clearly articulate a management philosophy, one couldn't know if their actions are consistent. Having already spent several years in management, I pondered my experiences and decided to sum it up in two words: "Respect and Autonomy." As a manager, I believe it is imperative to have Respect for each individual regardless of his or her job title. In addition, once given the expectations and resources to fulfill a job role, managers need to foster Autonomy within their staff as much as is feasible within each job description.

That MPH assignment was 14 years ago, and it was truly one of the most memorable and useful tasks that I was assigned during my post-graduate training. I have no doubt that each emerging manager needs to have a defined management philosophy that should be thought about often, and amended as necessary with increased experience.

If you are not at the table, you may be on the table

Early in my management career, I held leadership roles without clear job descriptions, and therefore had limited access to knowledge and information. Having learned that accurate information was imperative for success, I concluded that the best way to get information is to be in on the discussions. Offering to help and being willing to serve on committees are some of the easiest ways to get information quickly. In a large organization where there may be as much circulation of rumor as fact, it is useful to be part of multiple forums to best assess the accuracy of the available information. After participating in several arenas, I also learned that being at the table meant having a say in the destiny of my department. Without that participation, our needs were not taken into account and decisions made on our behalf often had unintended negative consequences. It is certainly better to be at the table than on the table!

Find your voice

Although a very successful student, I was rarely one to raise my hand. I was confident in what I knew, but never felt the need to demonstrate my expertise to others unless I was directly asked or challenged. This approach did not hamper my ability to graduate as valedictorian of my high school, but did negatively impact my success on hospital rounds, and was definitely not credibility-enhancing in management discussions. While I readily learned to contribute to clinical and middle management discussions, the development of my executive voice and presence was a more conscious endeavor.

Over the past 2 years, I have had the opportunity to engage an executive coach. Much of my work with her has been about finding my "executive voice" and learning to wield it. I first had to learn and accept that my current title and position comes with power—the power to question, to influence, and to act. To be effective in my job, it was imperative that I own this power and use it wisely, or someone else would, and perhaps not as judiciously. At this point, into my fourth year as Chief Operating Officer, I am comfortable speaking my mind in a variety of settings on a variety of topics. Aside from being more familiar with the topics and issues at hand and having the increased confidence that comes with experience, I have the comfort of owning my position and title. Where I once downplayed the significance of my executive position, I no longer feel apologetic about my administrative role. Instead, I embrace the possibilities of the unique contribution that I am able to make as a physician executive and use the opportunities to communicate effectively from a position of strength.

"Do something each day that scares you"

– Eleanor Roosevelt

While I don't do a scary thing every day, I do periodically seek out new challenges when I begin to feel comfortable in my primary job. This helps me stay at the top of my game, avoid complacency, and remain humble and honest with myself about how much more I still have to learn. Last year, for example, I joined the Board of Directors of a medical professional liability company. It was in a related field, but in an area that I knew almost nothing about. After a full day of board orientation, meeting with each member of the C-suite Executives, I gained a clear understanding of the strategic challenges facing the company. More importantly, I came to understand that the skills and knowledge I had acquired as a member of a successful senior management team translated well to another industry. While I still had to learn the specific technical content of the insurance industry, I already possessed the skills required for strategic planning, assessment of competition, understanding of information technology needs, and marketing and business development. Moreover, as a senior manager in my own organization, I had a greater understanding as to the separate and complementary responsibilities of the Board and Management, and what specific roles each should play to optimize the functioning of the other. Most importantly, I appreciated what the Board needs to leave to Management to operationalize and execute, and when the Board needs to be clear in its strategic planning and direction.

The gift of mentoring

To have a strong mentor is a gift. At several key times in my life, I've been fortunate to benefit from the guidance of a mentor. The willingness of someone experienced and well respected in their field to reserve personal time for me was greatly appreciated and needed. I used the opportunity to ask questions, to explore hypothetical situations, and simply to listen—to listen carefully and discern the pearls of wisdom born of challenges large and small; to understand that there is another way of approaching something. The best mentors have been people who offer concepts to consider and not rules to follow; a compass, not a map. Early in my career, it was harder to appreciate philosophical advice.

Sometimes it was easier to just have someone tell me what to do. It would have been easier, but clearly not better. I always learned more when I fully considered the points and counterpoints involved, made a decision for myself, and experienced the consequences.

As I have taken on the role of mentor myself, I recognize that the opportunity of mentoring is perhaps a greater gift because it is learning at a higher level. In fact, in the role of mentor I have learned as much if not more than I have as the mentee. This is likely because being a mentor necessitates greater introspection, personal accountability, and consistency of behavior. However, I could only function in this role after having had strong mentors who taught me what to expect.

Being a mentor is unlike any other relationship. It is different from being either a friend or a supervisor. As a friend, my primary role would be to support my friend's desire to make changes. As a supervisor, I am charged with keeping my employee accountable to stated responsibilities and provide additional opportunities for growth. The primary investment is in the individual as an employee, limited within the parameters of the organization's needs. As a mentor, my investment is in the individual as a person, the result of which may extend beyond the needs of the organization if the mentee is also an employee.

In my personal experience, the beginning of a mentoring relationship can be either a formal request for mentoring, or more frequently, the product of multiple informal conversations around aspirations. There is the recognition that there is a potential within the mentee to achieve something significantly beyond his or her current endeavors. This may have been something consciously or sub-consciously desired, but typically unspoken until that point.

Once identified, it is now up to the mentee to engage and decide whether this is a goal to pursue. If there is the agreement, then the relationship is set as I provide my commitment to nurture that potential to fruition, even if that ultimately results in the mentee taking a position in another organization. To me, the agreement is a key element because it advances the foundation of trust that is necessary for the mentorship to flourish. Without this trust, I will be unable to successfully challenge my mentee to reach outside of his or her comfort zone to gain new experiences, build confidence, and most importantly engage in honest self-assessments and further goal-setting. In addition, the explicit agreement assures that the goals represent an alignment with the mentee's desires, and not my personal goals for him or her to achieve. This conscious awareness and separation is needed so that there are no unrealistic or unspoken expectations at play that may result in misunderstandings or miscommunication. To be done well, mentoring is a slow and steady process, not to be rushed but readily cultivated.

I come to work to relax!

I have often joked that I come to work to relax. That's because my real life as wife and mother of four is far more demanding and challenging to manage than any project at work, no matter how difficult the issue. Early on, I felt guilty about being a working mother, worrying that the pursuit of my own career would equate on some level to neglecting my children, and that they would grow up either resenting it or feeling an element of loss.

Even as a child dreaming about my future, it was always a fantasy of working full-time and being an involved mother once I was home. There was never any doubt that I would not be working. And yet, when I had my first child during my chief resident year, I gave more thought to being a stay-at-home mother than I ever thought I would. I felt guilty about turning over her care to someone else. If not for the fact that I was obligated to return to my chief resident year, I might have pursued a longer maternity leave. For each child, the weeks leading up to the end of my maternity leave were the hardest. Those emotions did not lessen for subsequent children, even though I knew that it would work out well once the transition was made.

Reserved by nature, it was several years before I considered being candid about my internal conflicts in being a working mother. However, the experience of sharing with others allowed me to verbalize my own personal reality. I concluded that in many ways, I was a better mother when I was working. I appreciated my children more. I was able to focus on them more when I had been away. I treasured more the day-to-day achievements. I am sure I was more patient with them when I had not been there the whole day. And yet, the ultimate test of what I would choose if my career and motherhood met head-to-head came during a very inauspicious summer morning eight years ago.

I was at a routine prenatal ultrasound when we were told that our fourth child had a complex congenital heart defect. In the weeks that followed, through literature searches, consultation visits and long nights filled with uneasy thoughts and dreams, my husband and I eventually settled on a plan to have our son's delivery and subsequent surgery at a world-renowned university hospital that was out-of-state. Faced with an uncertain future that may not allow for out of home childcare, I carefully considered my career. I was frank with our CEO, our Chief Personnel Officer, and our Chief Medical Officer about the very real possibility that I might not be returning to work, and that it was even less likely that I could return to resume my role as the Site Medical Director of our largest clinic. They were incredibly supportive, exploring the option that the position be held in reserve for me by having an Acting Site Medical Director. I agreed, appreciative of their overwhelming support, and grateful for having an ideal job.

As I anticipated my last day at work before maternity leave, I imagined I would be emotional and maybe a bit conflicted. However, when that day arrived and I realized that I might be walking away from my career permanently, there was no ambivalence. In fact, I felt a great sense of peace. There was a remarkable clarity in my vision, knowing where I needed to be and what I needed to do. I knew then, that no matter how much I enjoyed my job, being a mother came first.

Two weeks later, our child was born. He had open heart surgery at 9 days old, and came home from the ICU at 3 weeks old. We were on a flight back home, all six of us, within 24 hours. I had very minimal contact with my practice in the early months, but as the situation improved, I started attending phone meetings during baby nap times, and slowly started to work on projects from home. At 7 months, my son started full-time daycare as I returned to work. It was then that I also started a support group for families affected by congenital heart issues, which continues to this day, over 7 years later. Within the group, we share a bond as heart families. Being on this journey together, rather than individually in isolation, makes all the uncertainty and challenges much more bearable.

I write this as our oldest is planning her freshman year at UC Berkeley, our second ready to start high school, our third due to start middle school, and our youngest looking forward to third grade. The search for work-life balance is an ever present and evolving process. I have come to realize that much of my guilt as a working mother was self-imposed and have come to understand that children who are cared for by loving adults will thrive in the environments in which they find themselves, even if it is not always in the company of parents. I devote as much time as I can to actively participate in their lives, whether in the classroom, on the sports field, or at the dining table over homework. But the best conversations are always had during my hours as a "chauffeur". That's when we discuss the compelling questions that reflect the most important issues in their lives at that moment. Being able to be present at those times has been priceless.

It is not always lonely at the top

Having worked in a variety of organizations, one topic of some controversy is whether it is acceptable to be personal friends with a direct report, and by extension, with those who report to them. There is no doubt that some level of personal engagement enhances work relationships, but should that extend to a personal friendship? In general, a level of professional friendliness is more than sufficient for a successful work relationship. And yet, if it is desired, I feel strongly that it is possible to have personal friendships at work, even in a management position. However, there needs to be an awareness of the inherent risk in being friends with your direct reports because you hazard the real or perceived loss of objectivity as it relates to that individual. Moreover, the subsequent decisions that are made may be subject to greater scrutiny or possible misinterpretation. This is a risk that can be largely eliminated by not pursuing a friendship, but it is not completely removed because there may be incorrect perceptions that arise of their own accord.

Still, I believe friendships can be successfully pursued if there is confidence in being able to handle the risks. For me, the friendship must not influence my ability to provide feedback, pursue accountability, impose disciplinary action, or assign resources or opportunities. I approach issues and consequences from a factual, principled basis. That is, I first examine the situation, whether positive or negative, for its objective elements. Then I determine the relevant consequences that need to be applied. These are based upon principles embodied within existing policies or guidelines or are extrapolated from precedence. In this approach, the specific individual, and thereby the relationship, is secondary to the decisions that need to be made.

These complex relationships do require that greater care and conscious awareness go into seemingly everyday decisions. The friendship should be neither secret nor flaunted, but publicly acknowledged when relevant. Social opportunities, especially those of general interest, should be offered equitably to all direct report peers whenever feasible. Some may consider this degree of effort more work than a friendship should entail, not worth the risks, or unwise to pursue. It may therefore be prudent for those individuals to avoid developing friendships at work. As for me, I have met many remarkable individuals in my days at work, and while I continue to navigate these relationships mindfully, I know that these friendships have enriched my life both personally and professionally and find all the effort quite worthwhile.

Maybe you can have it all

So the question remains, is it possible to have it all? I would like to believe that it is, but not always all at once. Aside from the basics of time management, prioritization, and organization, it comes down to some blind faith, a realization that I don't have to do it alone, and a good dose of personal forgiveness. It is the ability to recognize when some things are good enough and which elements demand flawless execution. It is the willingness to stay up late on more than a few nights when it is needed, not have a spotless house, and know when to walk away from the work for a little while in order to center myself. I am frequently asked how I stay so positive and keep from burning out. My answer has been the same over time. I trust my internal gauge as to whether I am having fun. If I am not, it is time to take a break and recharge.

Looking to the future

I am currently in my dream job, and I could easily see myself retiring from this position in the distant future. However, with the ever-changing health care landscape, I would not rule out the possibility of pursuing other opportunities if the need or possibility presented itself. In the more immediate future, I am interested in pursuing an MBA, to obtain formal business training. I will spend some time gaining more understanding about hospitals and health systems, as the future is likely to require greater involvement and understanding between different healthcare delivery entities. Along the way, I will continue to look for the fun in what I am doing and follow my internal compass of knowing when to chart a different course, if there is a need. I will continue to look for opportunities to do things that scare me and keep me from becoming complacent. Lastly, I look forward to learning from the wisdom of those more experienced, and welcome the opportunity to mentor others who may benefit from my own experiences and knowledge.

CHAPTER THIRTEEN

Pearls are a Woman's Necktie

by Grace Terrell, MD

I grew up in rural North Carolina in the 1960s, the oldest of four children. I was a classic tomboy, spending most of my free time playing outside with my brothers and cousins when I wasn't working in the garden, feeding the livestock, going to school and church, or watching favorite TV shows. My first years in school were stressful for me, because temperamentally I was different from the other girls. As a result I was picked on by the boys, and became disruptive in class. I dreaded report card days, when my all A record was inevitably spoiled by that D minus in conduct. Although the bullying I experienced in school was quite severe, as I gradually became more confident of my own talents and self-worth it actually made me fearless. Later, as a medical student and resident, behavior others would interpret as harassing or abusive just rolled right off my back.

Reading finally saved me from perpetual misery at school. I devoured books by the dozen and developed a love of reading that has remained an important part of my life. My parents knew they had their hands full with me, so they made sure I had lots of activities to keep me focused. Starting at age six, I participated in scouting, choral music, piano lessons, oil painting, and plays. Though not typical then, this was very much like the activity-filled lives of many children today. I even had my own horse, named Daisy. Since none of my other siblings liked to ride, some of my best memories are of my Dad and me riding our horses together.

The culture in which I grew up drew clear distinctions between the roles of girls and boys and I often felt uncomfortable with those traditionally assigned to women. I didn't want to learn to cook, sew, or homemaking and I didn't want to become a secretary, teacher, or nurse—the only careers I thought available to women. Although I had the highest grade point average in my class, I was told to learn to type. That way, "if I had to work", I could always get a job.

Prior to Title Nine, there were few sports opportunities for girls. I was jealous of my brothers' participation on baseball and football teams. I wanted to be an athlete, but year after year I was cut from the basketball team, the only sport open to girls at the time. Despite many hours of practicing alone, my petite and clumsy self couldn't seem to master the game. Luckily, I discovered running. In ninth grade I tried out for track and excelled, lettering in it. The following year, there were not enough girls trying out to form team, so I ran on the boys' team. I ran the mile and the 880. Every boy I beat would promptly quit the team as a matter of pride rather than wait to be cut. As a result, I was middle of the pack at the first of the season but dead last by the end.

As a young person, I began to become a student of human nature. This was in part a result of experiencing so much death in my people I was close to, including family. First my grandfather died of a cardiomyopathy at age 59. Not long after, my third grade school teacher died of metastatic breast cancer in the middle of the school year. My other grandfather died of coronary disease when I was in eighth grade and one of my grandmothers died of colon cancer when I was fifteen. My last grandparent died of a stroke when I was nineteen. My parents are only twenty and twenty-two years older than me. As I think back now, they had lost all four of their parents before they were forty. They were wrestling with all the issues of young adulthood while deeply grieving. In the midst of all that, they were able to create a family life that emphasized the moral imperative to make one's life meaningful in a loving and supportive environment. The message I heard from my mother, whose own life choices had been theoretically limited by economic circumstances was "you can do anything you want to do, Grace, so long as you set your mind to it." This existentialist message I have taken to heart.

Like Barack Obama, I graduated high school in 1979. This was the class that divided the baby boomer from generation X. I believe our values are boomer: i.e., focused on hard work, achievement, finding meaningfulness in our careers and life choices. But our circumstances are X-er: i.e., attending high school during recessionary, Watergate-driven cynical 70's, graduating college in the midst of the Reagan recession of 1983, entering our fifties after the 2007 crash. From a leadership perspective, this historical margin creates the possibility of a group of individuals who are simultaneously idealistic and cynical, hard working and somewhat self-centered. That juxtaposition allows a certain degree of conviction mixed with energy, perseverance, and caution that may be just what is necessary to lead us through our current national challenges.

In 1979, I won a Morehead scholarship to attend the University of North Carolina at Chapel Hill. At that point, the scholarship had only been open to females for three years. The scholarship allowed me to obtain an incredibly rich undergraduate education. During the summer months before college I participated in an Outward Bound program in Colorado. I got to ride a plane for the first time, and spent four weeks in the Rockies in a challenging physical and mental environment. Other summer experiences included working for a police department in California, a law firm in North Carolina, and, in 1982, during the Falklands War, working for the Liberal Whip's Office of the Parliament of Great Britain. In college I ran on the women's track team for a year and participated in Crew another year. Track turned me into a life-long runner. Choosing a major was difficult because I wanted to learn "everything". I ultimately majored in religion and English, with enough economics courses to nearly declare a third major.

More importantly, college is where I met the love of my life. Tim is the fifth of six children. Both his mother and father are physicians. Like me, he grew up in a large, close-knit family. We had both grown up on farms where we lived with grandparents in the same house. Our families were intensely committed to Democratic politics in an increasingly conservative state and equally involved in church—his were sixth-generation Quakers, mine were Southern Baptists. College for me included student government, track, and crew. For Tim it included managing the kitchen at his fraternity, delivering pizzas for Dominos, working as a camp counselor, exploring the new field of computer science with punch cards, algorithms, and programming. We both majored in religion, because it was the most intellectually comprehensive department in the university.

A week after we graduated in 1983 we married. In the midst of a recession, we had about five hundred dollars between us, no job, and liberal arts degrees in humanities. A year before, almost on a whim, I began thinking about medical school. The idea of taking a deep dive into the natural sciences, which I had not really studied since high school, with a career focused on helping people seemed appealing. Tim's mother, Dr. Eldora Terrell was a role model. She showed me such a life was possible. In an era in which women's choices were supposedly fixed, she had six children, practiced internal medicine, founded a clinic for uninsured patients in the community, took a public stand for integration in the Civil Rights era, was active in her church, serve as a medical director of a nursing home, a college board trustee, chief of staff of the hospital where she attended patients, and still managed to can green beans, make strawberry jelly, harvest asparagus, and ride horses to help with the cattle round-up on the weekends. Through her, I saw how the professional role of physician actually frees women from certain social constraints.

Ten days after graduating and three days after getting married I was in summer school studying physics. That wasn't the only course I had to take before applying to medical school. There were two physics courses, two organic chemistry courses, and some biology. Then I had to take the MCAT and do well in order to be accepted.

From 1983 to 1985 we lived in Richmond, Indiana while Tim pursued a Master's Degree in Quaker history at Earlham School of Religion. We had a three room cinderblock apartment in an undergraduate dormitory where I worked as Head Resident. My salary was three thousand dollars a year. We ate for free in the campus cafeteria. I thought it was the coldest place in the universe.

At age twenty-two, I found myself married to a creative, idealistic, and definitely unfocused man, working in a job where I was responsible for students only a few years younger than myself. They challenged me, insulted me, and generally pursued their own agendas. They didn't know that I had a recent "grand past" as a Morehead scholar, intern to Parliament, and UNC varsity athlete. To them, I was either the person who let them into their dorm room when they lost their key, the one from whom they hid their marijuana, or the person who was supposed to settle their roommate complaints. For intellectual enrichment I took a "wives' course" on John Updike at the School of Religion. It was awful: faculty wives crocheting and talking about their children's preschool experiences.

Tim was trying to find himself and I was trying not to lose myself. I focused upon those science courses at the college that I needed for medical school. Fortunately I could take these virtually for free as part of my employment. In addition, I decided to expand my general knowledge base. First, I found a Cliff's Notes pamphlet and looked at all the great books listed on the back page. Then I started from the A's to the Z's and read each work of literature, from "Absalom, Absalom" on down the alphabet. After that I read all the works of philosophy I could locate including all of Hegel, all of Kant, all of Kierkegaard, and so on.

I told myself I was doing this before I went to medical school because then I wouldn't have time to read for pleasure. In retrospect, though, I was probably depressed. Training and running a triathlon finally got me out of my funk. I took the MCAT, interviewed and applied for several medical schools. I was accepted at Duke and entered in 1985.

Tim and I traded places in the fall of 1985. Suddenly I was the medical student, with purpose and focus, and he was looking for a job. He worked as a bartender in the Duke faculty lounge for a bit, and finally landed a job counseling Native American high school students, helping them get into college through the North Carolina Commission of Indian Affairs. For the first two years we scraped by on his $13,500 a year salary. Then we decided we just had to have a baby.

Katy was born at the end of my third year of medical school. I took eight weeks off, then did my fourth year "in reverse", taking the sub-internships at the end of the fourth year rather than at the beginning. The year Katy was born Tim decided to return to school for a master's degree in the burgeoning new field of computer science. He took all of his classes on Tuesdays and Thursdays so he could be home with the baby on the other days. On Tuesdays and Thursdays, my sister, a freshman at UNC drove over to Durham to watch the baby, while Tim drove over to NC State University to take his classes. After I graduated from medical school, I stayed at Duke Medical Center an extra year and did an internship in pathology, reasoning that without night call I could be with the baby at home giving Tim time to finish his degree.

My year as a pathology intern still seems surreal. Like many working mothers I felt the pangs of guilt every morning as I left my daughter at home. It didn't matter that her father and aunt were available as primary care givers. Katy walked early, talked early, and was like a little Tasmanian devil full of energy. I hated missing any part of her development, although her irregular sleeping and eating patterns kept us all perpetually exhausted. I spent my days doing surgical and autopsy pathology. The autopsies on fetuses and children were particularly difficult for me. I still remember how I felt entering the autopsy suite to view one particular case. The little girl was almost the same age as my Katy, her body in a nightgown, still clutching a teddy bear.

Like many internships of that era, the pathology department at Duke was not a particularly warm environment. Because the program directors knew I did not intend to remain in pathology as a specialty, they focused their mentoring energies elsewhere. When some of the physicians learned of my plan to practice general internal medicine, I began to experience discrimination for the first time. Duke was not primary care friendly. One professor told me that I should leave and find some primary care program in a community setting, that as a "real" academic institution, there was no place for a generalist at Duke.

That year while in the surgical suite, I accidentally severed the artery and nerve to my left index finger on a formalin-hardened surgical specimen. The injury required hand surgery. For eight weeks while the re-anstamosis healed I was unable to cut surgical specimens. When I returned to work the day after my surgery, an upper level resident yelled at me for a good thirty minutes, making it clear that my injury was going to make life difficult for the other pathology interns. The department administrator was equally unsympathetic, his only concern that this might bring OSHA down on the department.

Once Tim finished his degree, we knew we needed to make a change. I was accepted into the primary care track in internal medicine at NC Baptist Hospital in Winston-Salem. I completed my pathology internship on June 29th, 1990, and began my second internship July 1. That was the start of the second craziest year of my life. We were living with Tim's parents, in High Point, NC about twenty miles from Winston Salem. Tim got a job in Public Health Sciences in research computing at the medical school. Our household was not exactly mainstream America. We had four generations, including Tim's ninety-four year old grandmother, my busy internist mother-in-law and father-in-law, Tim, me and Katy, the quintessential "terrible two" year old. The four dogs in the house added to the chaos. Still, it was wonderful having the security of two salaries for the first time after eight years of marriage.

Like every other medical intern, I rotated through cardiology, heme-onc, general medicine, emergency medicine, and the other specialties with every second or third night call. I do not remember that time as being difficult or abusive. I was excited to finally learn my craft in a residency environment that was both rigorous and supportive. I developed a very close relationship with Dr. Bryant Kendrick, a chaplain at the medical center who managed the internal medical primary care track. He became my real mentor, helping me process my continued "strangeness": we focused upon medical ethical issues; the excitement engendered by the Clinton era anticipated health care reform, and the spiritual wholeness of the doctor-patient experience.

After fourteen months of living with Tim's parents, we had saved enough for a down payment to purchase our first house. It was on a wooded lot with a stream, a tree house, a swing set, and an elementary school and playground next door. We balanced our roles as young parents and professionals, began paying off our student loans, and spent our free time together hiking, parenting, exercising, and keeping up this new house.

In 1993, seven months pregnant with my second daughter, Robyn, I completed my residency and began private practice with my in-laws. I took my medical boards that September, before promptly going into labor. The next eight weeks were some of the sweetest of my life. I took maternity leave and was able to walk Katy to the neighborhood school for her first days of kindergarten. I also got to spend some very quiet and special time with my new little girl.

Although as grandparents, my in-laws were both interested in the welfare of their new granddaughter, as medical practice partners they were equally eager for my return to work. This was the period when primary care started to lose status and get slogged by the economic forces of managed care. Our once a week call meant covering seven internists, three nursing homes, and unassigned hospital cases. These were also the days before hospitalists and before nurse triage. The paradigm was still for the internist to be the center of all activity in the middle of the medical universe, despite the degradation of both reimbursement and status. It was far more brutal in many respects than my residency, but also more rewarding. The intensity of the experiences with patients in the office, the hospital, and the nursing home in that era has been unsurpassed. It was comprehensive and I had been trained to be effective in a multitude of settings. In areas where I had not, the forty-year experience of my father-in-law and mother-in-law filled in the gaps left in my training. It helped me understand the real role of physicians: to listen, to act, help, to heal.

About six months after I had joined my in-laws' private practice, administration at High Point Regional Hospital where I admitted patients, began discussions about the creation of a PHO (physician hospital organization) as a response to anticipated changes in the health care environment from managed care. The chief-of-staff, Dr. Al Hawks, gave a passionate speech about the need for collaboration and cooperation and a steering committee of seven was formed. The three specialists and three primary care physicians nominated to form the steering committee were all established male medical staff members.

Almost as an afterthought, my father-in-law nominated me. Over the course of the next eighteen months, we met every Thursday night, sometimes until one or two o'clock in the morning, to create what ultimately became Cornerstone Health Care. Most of us were junior partners in our practices. Because we were young and less established in the community, we were more willing to be reckless. We figured out our governance and income distribution, and began developing a culture based less on autonomy and more on collaboration. We also focused on investing in information, technology, and advanced models of care delivery.

Cornerstone Health Care was established October 1, 1995 from the merger of sixteen practices in High Point, NC. Seventeen years later I am its chief executive officer and have been so for the past twelve years. During that time, I have seen my daughters grow to young adults, my in-laws retire from medical practice and my practice merge with two other Cornerstone internal medical practices to become the first NCQA recognized level three Physician Practice Connection Medical Home in our state. Cornerstone has grown from the original sixteen practices in High Point, to seventy-three locations throughout the Piedmont Triad region of North Carolina, with over three hundred providers practicing in ten separate hospitals that are part of six separate health systems. Our company's focus is to be the model for physician-led health care in America. We are committed to transform our model from a volume-based system to one that is value-based, leading our market in innovative approaches to a sustainable twenty-first century health care delivery system.

My Message:

The story I have written here is not the one I expected to write. It is deeply personal and one that speaks to many elements of my life that are not directly pertinent to my day-to-day role as a physician executive. I have not discussed in detail my twelve years experience as chief executive officer or my greater than twenty years as a practicing physician in terms of lessons learned that might help other women physicians considering a career in medical management. Instead, I have decided to share my story within the context of my complex roles as daughter, mother, wife, and daughter-in-law because I believe it is these roles that help define how women are viewed as professionals and the special skills they bring to their leadership responsibilities.

We are at the beginning of what I expect will be the single fastest transformation of any industry in U.S. history. Physician leadership in health care during this transformation is crucial and the health care delivery system transformation will be an enormous opportunity for women. But the relative lack of women in leadership roles in health care currently needs to be understood and addressed.

I would suggest that one approach to addressing this discrepancy is through the language of archetypes as articulated by Carl Jung. Jung theorized that archetypes are symbolic figures hardwired into our unconsciousness. He focused upon the archetypes of hero, father, mother, temptress, witch, villain, wise old woman (or man), and innocent, ingrained in our collective unconsciousness as identified in myths across cultures and times. Unlike men, most of the female archetypes are characterized by relationships that adhere to traditional social roles (mother, daughter, grandmother, sister). Although men are also represented in archetypes based upon traditional social roles (father, son, grandfather, brother), there are some strong male archetypes based on the relationship between man and society. These are the roles of hero and villain, both of which are external to the family. The hero is focused more upon saving the group, defending the weak and innocent, administering justice. The villain is his foil.

Our country's future success depends upon our ability to transform our health care delivery system to one that is equitable, affordable, and effective. That transformation will require leadership from many individuals who have neither prepared for nor expected to play these critical roles. For women is it crucial that we understand that effective leaders learn the language of leadership and master it. Using Jung's paradigm, we need to appreciate how we are perceived in various situations in order to discern how a particular female gender archetype might impact our message. By listening to the language used by others we can create the situational story in which our role is played. Then we can choose which voice to use in order to be most effective leaders.

The *grandmother voice* is the storytelling voice. It is particularly useful when giving a presentation, as the human mind is designed to retain information it hears from stories. For physicians, a story about a patient that teaches a lesson and evokes empathy can be a very powerful tool. In the working world, the *mother voice* can be dangerous. It can be perceived as both loving and scolding, and should be used with caution. On the other hand, the *sister voice* is powerful because it is collaborative. The connotations of sisterhood eliminates inappropriate sexual overtones and its implied equal status in the sibling relationship can positively impact team building.

Women tend to overuse the *daughter voice*. Female subordinates often find the daughter role to be a safe relationship with male bosses/mentors because it may diminish sexual tension. However, this is a problem when attempting to transition to a leadership role. Beware of language in which sexual allusion are used in descriptions of women. The *temptress/prostitute* archetypes are universal and powerful, but not appropriate within the context of leadership. Likewise, the *domineering woman/bitch* role is dangerous. Some women avoid leadership roles because they fear being depicted within this context. The most enigmatic role for women is that of *witch*. The witch role is powerful, but frightening, because it is a role contextualized around female power that is outside of the standard male dominant cultural context. Powerful men may rely upon the language of the warrior/hero archetype as the context for their effective leadership, but being perceived as powerful using the witch archetype is generally a problem for women in leadership roles.

As leaders, women need to pay attention to the language in which you are speaking and the language in which others speak to you. Pay attention to the subtle messages of clothing, body language, and underlying archetypes in the language of colleagues. Choose the voice with which you speak and the language with which you organize your leadership roles. Think about those symbols that project power. Leadership is an existential construct based upon social roles, language, and archetypal understandings that constitute the deep wisdom written into the human experience. We ARE tomboys, sisters, mothers, daughters, grandmothers, temptresses, bitches and witches. To be leaders we must also be authentic. I do not believe authentic leadership for women is found within a neutered male heroic archetype. It rises out of our own experiences. Pearls are a woman's necktie.

MANAGED CARE
For Profit and Not-For-Profit

CHAPTER FOURTEEN

A Continuing Search for Challenge

by Christine A. Petersen, MD, MBA

The career of a medical manager can begin in many ways and take many paths. My thirty year journey has been satisfying and challenging, both professionally and personally. My early career was one of numerous relocations which provided me with expansion of my medical management experience and lessons in adapting to different management styles, reporting relationships and job responsibilities. For my young children, these moves meant adapting to new schools, new friends and ever changing nannies and childcare givers. I spent ten years as CMO and Vice President of Medical Affairs at Sierra Health Services in Las Vegas, Nevada before choosing retirement when the corporation was sold to United Healthcare. Instead of ending my management career, I transitioned to a new leadership role as head of my own health care consulting practice. Unlike working within various managed care organizations, consulting brought its own set of challenges but it has allowed me to utilize all the skills and experience I have been fortunate enough to obtain over the years and to continually expand my professional network.

I am a board certified internist and had a private practice in Grand Junction Colorado. In 1983 I was asked to become the first full time medical director of Rocky Mountain HMO. Although I was intrigued by the idea, I initially said no. I couldn't imagine leaving my practice and patients. Four months later, I was telling my patients that my move out of practice was only temporary and I would return to private practice in two years.

I had absolutely no experience as a medical manager other than participation in HMO committees. As I started to perform my job I realized that I had no management or business tools other than intuitive ones. My CEO and mentor supported my decision to join the American College of Physician Executives and take Seminars I and II. What an eye opener. Suddenly the lights went on and the pieces began to fall into place. I was hooked. I developed a detailed business plan for myself which focused on enhancing my medical management experience, obtaining expanded responsibilities and positioning for advancement.

In 1985, FHP, Inc, then a primarily staff model HMO, was expanding into the IPA arena in new geographic areas. I accepted a position as Medical Director for the new Arizona Region. The challenges were incredible and the experience invaluable. I had the opportunity to start the medical department from scratch, help create and manage thirteen separate IPAs, introduce the specialists to capitation and interface with all the other providers required for a complete network. We applied for and received a Medicare Risk contract, another set of challenges and opportunities! Two and a half years later, we had 50,000 members, started our staff model overlay and began our Tucson expansion.

My next move was to Corporate headquarters in Southern California as part of the Medical Affairs team. I completed my MBA to help advance my career and broaden my business training. My children and I loved living in California, but I really wanted more operational responsibility so when an opportunity came up with FHP in Utah we went for it. In addition to my responsibility for Medical Affairs I had P and L responsibility for our large dental, optical, and pharmacy operations. We were also in the final architectural drawing phase for our hospital construction and that was a fabulous challenge. There were so many time sensitive tasks from medical staffing to policies and procedures and everything in between. Three years later the hospital was opened and the first surgical procedure performed. I was then offered a position back at Corporate as Vice President of Medical Affairs so the children and I moved back to California. During that time I was responsible for medical informatics, medical policies and procedure, medical management education, training and recruiting. The role was challenging, but I really wanted to get back into the direct operations. When I was recruited to Prudential Health Care to work in Southern Group Operations in Atlanta we were on the road again.

This position came with lots of travel throughout the South East and opportunities to meet and work with many different and talented people. It also gave me the chance to work for a very large company with a national presence. After fourteen months in Atlanta I was asked to become the National Director for Utilization Management with responsibility for forty-five plans. I was tasked to develop the business plan for Medicare Risk contracting expansion. I lived in Atlanta, but also maintained an office in New Jersey. If I thought I was traveling before it didn't hold a candle to this. Every week I was in either a different city or in New Jersey.

I must admit it was brutal, but worth every minute. My network was really expanded at this point and by this time I had acquired experience in almost every area in the world of medical management.

The key word was "almost". I hadn't yet been a Chief Medical Officer. When the opportunity came up to become the CMO for Sierra Health Services in Las Vegas of course I couldn't resist. The fact that many of my former FHP colleagues were working there made the transition relatively easy. The position brought a whole new world of very different experiences. Although I had no direct line operational responsibility, I loved my job. I interfaced with the press, community leaders, and participated on the Leadership Council at AHIP. Together with my team, I helped to set medical policy, new technology review, and interfaced with legislative issues. As we purchased operations, I participated with numerous due diligence efforts. Ten years after I arrived, we were purchased by United Health Care.

Although I " retired", I was never one to resist a challenge. While I was at Sierra I worked with a group to start a clinic in Tanzania. After "retirement" I was able to spend more time there, hire and train staff, see lots of patients and help with fundraising. We now have a clinic, a small hospital, birthing unit, surgery unit, maternal and childcare unit and dental. Optical will arrive soon. After the sale to United Health Care I worked with a group of physicians in Las Vegas to help set up a Free clinic that would serve the needs of the uninsured, I continue as Vice President of the Board. I serve on other non profit boards related to health care and stay active in the professional community.

So what didn't I have? Business cards. The answer to that was to set up a consulting company with myself as principal. I was spending time with my grandchildren, traveling and just enjoying myself and never planned to start of a substantial business. However, if you maintain your networks, your contacts will find you. So I am now in the wide world of consulting and dealing with new challenges.

Lessons I have learned in my career:

- Seek challenges

- Develop and maintain your professional network

- Keep open to moves to new geographic areas

- Respect your colleagues

- Mentor your staff

- Give back to your community

- Have fun

CHAPTER FIFTEEN

A Managed Care Journey:
Learning from Yourself and Others

by Susan Elizabeth Ford, MD, MBA

I participated in the 1995 version of "Women in Medicine and Management". Sixteen years later, I truly appreciate the opportunity to once again reflect on my career. By sharing my secrets to success, I hope to inspire the next generation of women in medicine. My life choices thus far have been sculpted by my ever-evolving visions, expectations, and experiences that have led me from clinician to medical manager.

I'd like to begin by describing those personal characteristics and propensities that have been instrumental in my decision making over the years. These will provide the reader with a framework to understand the choices I have made along my career path. First, I am very focused. One of my most important life goals is to make positive contributions in everything I do, including my work. Second, I like process. I enjoy improving upon the status quo. Third, I love learning and intellectually challenging myself. Fourth, like many physicians, I am pragmatic and persistent, but unlike some, I also possess intuition, which drives me to think creatively and helps with planning long-term strategies and goals. From my vantage point, setting goals is fundamental to achieving a successful and rewarding career in any field.

At the age of 12, I set a rather large goal for myself. I decided to become a physician "because I liked science and working with people." This pre-teen goal turned into both my lifelong career and passion. It required discipline, hard work, and self-motivation—even when times got tough. Having unwavering faith in my abilities, I turned adversity into self-motivation. This proved to be a prescription for success in my life. I was valedictorian in high school and went off to medical school after only two years of college.

After attending evening Family Practice club meetings as a med student at the University of Maryland Medical School, I made the decision to become a Family Practitioner. It made perfect sense. I enjoyed all of my rotations in medical school equally and did not want to give up any area of medicine in order to specialize. At that time, Family Practice was considered a brand new specialty requiring a rigorous, three year residency. However, not everyone appreciated the breadth of knowledge required of those choosing that field. Many of my colleagues and professors urged me to specialize in a more narrow area, telling me that I was too "smart" to be a GP. I disagreed, deciding not to take their advice.

At this point in my career, I was committed to clinical practice. I hadn't given any real thought to medical management although I definitely had an interest in the technologic advances made in medicine and was concerned with how poorly these advances had been implemented in the general population. Whenever I was bored in class, I would find myself doodling and coming up with ways to redesign anything to do with healthcare—from reconfiguring delivery systems, to office layouts, to brainstorming better procedural methods.

In 1977, I completed my Family Practice residency and passed the specialty board exam. In my last year, acting as chief resident, I developed an interest in teaching and working with residents. I became involved in Family Medicine training programs and participated in a fellowship in the Faculty Development Program at Jefferson Medical College in Philadelphia. The fellowship covered many areas that were useful not only for teaching, but for medical management. Topics included adult learning theory, behavioral learning, budget development, counseling skills, curriculum development, management by objectives, and broad evaluation skills. We also worked on audit and performance feedback skills. There are many similarities between teaching and managing skills. In retrospect, I found that the fellowship was a great forum for learning generic medical management skills. After completion of the program, I remained at Jefferson as the coordinator for the Faculty Development Program.

While working at Jefferson Medical College, one of the residents introduced me to a book-lovers' club for single people. To make a long story short, I met my husband, who was living in the San Francisco Bay area. Because he let me choose which coast to live on when we married, we moved to San Francisco where I joined the Family Practice residency program in San Jose, California. There, I participated in the usual duties of residency faculty members, including teaching and supervision in the outpatient center. I had the opportunity to sit on several medical staff committees at the hospital. I also gave presentations to residents about the business side of practice including explaining different medical practice settings, such as Health Maintenance Organizations (HMOs). Through the process of developing lectures and training materials for residents, I became extremely interested in HMOs. I collected copious information about managed care and set up several job interviews.

My experiences in San Jose led me to a position with CIGNA Healthplan in Dallas. My position was actually three separate roles in one: practicing physician, chairman of Family Practice, and Chief of Staff of a health care center. Tough demanding, the job proved to be very useful in my growth as a medical manager. It was a natural fit—the organization needed a Family Practice department developed, and I wanted to learn about HMOs. Since this HMO health plan was in its infancy, it provided an excellent opportunity to learn how all the elements of an HMO fit together into a functioning system. During this time, I also had the chance to open and develop one of the centers as Chief of Staff. I participated actively on quality committees, and eventually was asked to assume the position of Associate Medical Director for Quality Assurance. In that role, I took my first major step into medical management.

Up to this point, my transition from clinical practice to medical management had consisted of gradually increasing administrative involvement. I always enjoyed problem solving with others to improve the big picture, but this was the first time in my career that my job became half administrative. I found that I really loved medical management, and felt that I could have a bigger impact by pursuing this career path rather than seeing individual patients. I became a member of the American Academy of Medical Directors, now the American College of Physician Executives, and attended two Physician in Management seminars.

Although I thoroughly enjoyed my experiences in Texas, after four years in the Lone Star State, my husband reminded me of my promise to move back to the West Coast if it provided better job opportunities for him. It was then that I realized achieving great success in life means more than having a distinguished career. It also means compromise and balance to ensure a happy, healthy relationship on the home front.

At the time we relocated to California, CIGNA had no Medical Director openings, so I found one with a small HMO. In addition to medical management, the position provided some exposure to various business departments within the organization. My responsibilities included medical department staffing, budgeting, utilization management, and quality assurance for a network with 29,000 patients. I also managed optometry, podiatry, mental health, medical operations, and home health. Since the HMO was relatively small, I had plenty of opportunity to interact with the finance and business departments. I also learned, by way of the school of hard knocks, how to handle situations that conflicted with my personal ethics.

It was at this point when I learned—or re-learned, if you will—a critical life lesson. It is important to be comfortable and enthusiastic about your organization's goals and ethics. Those goals and ethics should align with yours. The man or woman you report to should be someone you respect, someone of good conscience who will always do the right thing. Never work for organizations that just want to use power or that do not clearly add value to the big picture. Remember this: Power, like information, must be used appropriately and shared to produce optimal results.

As a physician manager, it is particularly important that the organization appreciate and support your "physician" expertise in advocating for high-quality health care. Health care advocacy is ideally a natural position for all physicians. For a health organization, it must be a key element in any well-balanced business equation. We, as medical managers, must preserve the professional principles of medicine in our work and be clear about our goals and visions and be single-minded in their pursuit.

In 1989, I passed the American Board of Medical Management certifying exam. Following this accomplishment, I took a position as Staff Medical Director for CIGNA Healthplan near Los Angeles. In that role, I had a broad range of responsibilities, including utilization management, provider network, hospital contracting, home health, and 24-hour telephone triage for 380,000 managed care patients. In addition, I had oversight for the areas that handled medical case management, medical claim review, medical social work, medical benefits interpretations, and technology assessment. While at CIGNA, I earned a Master of Business Administration (MBA) from the Executive MBA Program at the University of Southern California.

The degree, combined with my years of management experience, opened up many new doors. I worked for Aetna as the Market Medical Director for Aetna Health Plans in Los Angeles; for United Health Care in Nebraska; and for provider-owned MCOs in Oklahoma and New Mexico. In each position I gained valuable skills, but chose to move on for various reasons: family, growth opportunities, and intuition that a job change would be best for my career.

It is my hope that my current role as Medical Director for Amerigroup New Mexico will be my position for many years to come because it fits me well, and I don't plan to retire as long as I am able to work. The content of my job is varied and constructive and the work philosophy is well-balanced. Amerigroup's business is Medicaid and Medicare, but in New Mexico, we also have a Coordinated Long-Term Services (CoLTS) Program dedicated to the needs of seniors and people with disabilities. CoLTS integrates medical services with home and community based care, serving those with disabilities in a manner that promotes independent living. This position challenges and excites me. It involves a never-ending array of interesting problem-solving that results in improved health outcomes for our members.

Over the years I have learned that one gains credibility and competence from real experience and accomplishments, and I am incredibly proud of the various work experiences I have had. Each experience has challenged me to learn and try new things. While continuing education is integral in our field, I firmly believe exposure to different situations and actual life experience is essential to success. I have experienced many types of management, planning and strategy development and organizational structures, and have seen strengths and weaknesses in each situation. I have had many successes and failures and have learned from them all. I encourage you to take chances, dare to dream, set goals and find a work life balance that is right for you. As far as mentoring (giving or receiving), I have been egalitarian in terms of person, gender, or professional credentials. It's important to be open-minded and always remember that one can learn from others or mentor others at any time or place.

Here are some parting thoughts on making goals a reality:

Important Skills and Traits to Develop:

- Creativity and flexibility—change is a given and essential element of life

- Negotiation skills—and conflict resolution

- Contribution—as "How do I bring something to the interaction?"

- Creating value for the whole system—ask "Is this good for the whole or just my compartment?"

- Teamwork and collaboration

- Enthusiasm—be positive and don't get cynical or negative, get people enthusiastic about work

- Persistence

- Prioritization—protect your time and control perfectionistic tendencies; close your office door when it is necessary to concentrate

- Learning to lose, risk, try, learn—welcome opportunities

- Forgetting past inequities—they just demean and slow one down

Some Skills for Working on One's Career Development (Self-Mentoring):

- Brainstorm and write down ideas, goals, and specific steps. Then, get them organized and prioritized. Putting your ideas on paper in an organized way helps move from thoughts and ideas to reality.

- Always have a clear idea of your main goals, tasks, and time frames for both the short run and the long run.

- Mentally practice scenarios. Visualize positive and successful situations. Don't be too humble. Mentally practice how you will proceed in specific situations. Imagine certain interactions in detail or go through mock dialogues with a trusted person. View yourself positively while you do this.

- Study your own experience and observe others to improve yourself.

CHAPTER SIXTEEN

The 'Other' Side

by Deborah E. Hammond, MD

In the middle of a memorable phone conversation with a surgeon in 1988 regarding the lack of approval for an elective procedure, the decibels suddenly decreased and the surgeon's tone shifted to one of open questioning. "How did you get this job? What do you have to do to get this job? I have been thinking about a change. Would you recommend this type of job?" After a few seconds of stunned readjustment on my part, we went on to have a very pleasant conversation covering these questions. We then completed our less than pleasant discussion concerning the lack of approval for the surgical procedure.

I related this story in the original "Women in Medicine and Management" monograph published 17 years ago because it had reaffirmed in my mind that the role of the professional medical manager is deeply involved in the running of health care organizations. In 1995 the medical manager role had already changed from a predominately end of career position to an option as an independent career path. That's even truer today.

Doing it Over

Now with the luxury of almost two more decades of experience, I am asked if I would do it all again. The answer is an emphatic "yes". Yes, even if I were just starting out in 2012 facing the implementation of the Patient Protection and Affordable Care Act (ObamaCare) rather than 1980 when I began my medical management career by volunteering to become a section leader at a group model health maintenance organization (HMO) in Suffolk County, New York.

So how does a person, especially a female physician, find or create the opportunities to take advantage of this option? An exploration of the path I took, the lessons I learned, and the skills that I believe are paramount to job satisfaction and job success may be helpful. My present position did not evolve from a pre-planned scheme. I came to this role using an ongoing process of defining and redefining my professional goals, of including the roles desired, of being open to and acting on opportunities to learn, of seeking out mentors to help guide me, of taking risks and trying new things, and, finally of actively identifying management and leadership skills that need improvement.

Professional Beginnings

My career in management began when I agreed, at the age of 16, to be a lead counselor for a summer day camp for kids. It was my first experience in the need for teamwork. Only years later did I realize that individual efforts account for a small portion of success in management. The team determines success!

My next lessons occurred during my college years. Each summer an anesthesiologist in Chicago and close family friend, hired me to fill in for vacationing support staff of an anesthesia department in a large teaching hospital. I acted as receptionist, secretary, library research assistant, and, most important, surgery scheduling clerk. I learned that real power and control lies in the hands of associates at the front line. The ability to hold sway over who obtains the 7 a.m. start times and back-to-back slots was a heady experience. As a dividend, I received a further lesson. Over time, nice guys (or gals) finish first. While a powerful surgeon could pull strings or, more commonly, rant and rave to get a preferred slot, it was the doctors who always went out of their way to be pleasant to the clerks (in some cases plying us with donuts) who consistently got the best times and preferred rooms. Use of position, title, or level in the organization to get people to act was at best an inconsistent and damaging tool.

My professional career in management began during Internal Medicine postgraduate training at Montefiore Hospital at the University of Pittsburgh. I supervised a five-week general medicine inpatient training period for a group of medical students and interns. This is an experience that male and female residents share equally in their early careers. While not formally recognized (the first formal recognition is commonly the chief resident position), this supervisory role should be used as the first step to building management skills for those interested in such a career. It is an opportunity to learn how to prioritize, distribute work, organize schedules, tutor and teach, and decide on who can be empowered to make certain decisions. (As an aside, I would suggest that graduate training leaders reading this include a formal evaluation of management skills for each resident and fellow).

My next most valuable lesson came from my first mentor, the Chief of the Department of Internal Medicine. He was an amazing person, able to deflate a pompous medical professional with a mere glance. One night, while covering the hospital, I was called to a cardiac arrest on the "gold coast" floor. A private duty nurse had been caring for the patient and in the midst of the chaos, I banished her from the room. In my mind, she had no idea what she was doing. The next day, I was called to the Chief's office. He first offered me tea and then in a calm way asked how publicly throwing the nurse out of the room helped the patient. With that one question, my defense crumbled. I knew he was right; it didn't help the patient. Lesson learned: The end does not justify the means, and the means can significantly hinder your success.

Real Jobs

My first formal management position happened quite by accident. I was in practice with a not-for-profit multi-specialty group on Long Island, New York, seeing a majority of HMO patients and a minority of indemnity fee-for-service patients. As a woman in practice in the early '80s, I attracted many older women who had been "waiting for a female doctor". I enjoyed the role of practicing Internist immensely, especially the aspect of continuity of care, something that was lacking in my medical school and postgraduate training. The HMO's adherence to preventive care for all members and the lack of financial barriers to obtaining high-quality health care for my patients fit my concept of providing accessible health care to all.

When the Chief of the Department of Medicine left, I assumed that an experienced administrator would be asked to assume the role, but the Medical Director came to me. After a brief period of consideration, I took the position. The lesson here was: don't be afraid to take risks. My first task (and nightmare) was to determine scheduling for Thanksgiving, Christmas, Hanukkah, and New Year's. The previous Chief had left little documentation. Each person claimed they had worked all the previous holidays. Remember, whatever the decision, you can't make everyone happy. That's a particularly difficult lesson for women to learn. I know I have an innate wish to please that cannot exist in full concert with the roles of effective manager and leader. However, it is important to be able to explain your reasons for the decision in the context of the overall vision of the organization, to demonstrate fairness, and to lack favoritism. In this case, I scheduled myself for Christmas and pointed out that care had to be provided, asking who wanted to work which holiday.

During this period, I began to work on quality assurance, utilization management, and associate training projects in the hospital and group practice setting. It is important to seek out these kinds of extracurricular opportunities. They provide opportunities to hone technical skills, to network, and to build a management résumé prior to your first formal management position.

Before starting this job, I had negotiated a year's leave of absence, unpaid, for future child bearing and rearing activities. Unless you are convinced that you will never want children, discuss and confirm maternity and child care benefits prior to taking any position. During my leave, following the birth of my daughter, my husband and I decided to leave New York for Oklahoma.

I returned to work as a volunteer instructor in ambulatory adult medicine at the Tulsa Medical College, University of Oklahoma. This allowed me to network, learn about practice opportunities, and be in the right place at the right time. Blue Cross and Blue Shield of Oklahoma was looking for an experienced managed care doctor to help start its first IPA capitated HMO. Because of the controversial nature of the project, physician leaders living in Oklahoma had turned down the Medical Director position. It was the early 1980s, and managed care was a controversial and undesired opportunity for the Oklahoma physician community. I decided to take a leap and move into full-time medical management. Once again, don't be afraid to take risks.

Here, I met my next mentor and my first non-physician boss. His unique approach was to demonstrate empathy and involvement to each and every associate. One particular crisis management issue exemplifies the value of his approach. Claims were behind, exacerbated by rapid membership growth. Claims associates were demoralized, and the manager position was unfilled. When I arrived at work on a Saturday morning, my boss asked me to help pay claims. It was a great experience. The associates were astonished and energized by the sight of our pitching in. Demonstrating that you are willing to walk in another person's shoes is a powerful team-building exercise.

In addition to building management skills, I was able to link with other Blue Cross and Blue Shield Medical Directors. Networking provided me with invitations to visit HMOs for in-depth sharing of best practices and of lessons learned. Networking provided me with peers who had gone through the same struggles as I had and who were a sympathetic sounding board. Networking provided me with my next job.

While in this position, I was also given the opportunity to serve as a consultant to the Federal Office of HMO, reviewing and scoring applications for federal HMO qualification. This allowed me to view best practices, meet industry leaders, and learn about the diversity of the managed care industry while honing my skills in consultation, analysis, and auditing. Advice: Locate part-time consulting opportunities, such as with the National Committee on Quality Assurance and the Joint Commission on Accreditation of Healthcare Organizations.

My next position came about when a Medical Director mentioned me (without my knowledge) as a potential candidate for a Regional Medical Director role with Prudential. I first turned down the position, but a subsequent interview with the new Vice President of Medical Services convinced me that this position was a risk worth taking. I had a new mentor in my new boss and a new role as a staff Medical Director supporting nine managed care operations. I was given opportunities to learn beyond the field of managed care. These included the methodology of life and health insurance underwriting, the handling of indemnity or traditional medical insurance administration, marketing to prospective national clients, running large-scale associate training programs, and the basic tenets of contract law and proactive risk management.

Once again, I let my boss and others know that I wanted to try new things. An invaluable experience was being placed on the team that transitioned 236,000 employees and dependents from an indemnity health care policy to a point-of-service managed care benefit plan in 14 locations.

Within a year, I was offered the position of Vice President of Medical Services, responsible for clinical leadership and oversight of both the managed care and the indemnity businesses. This was the most complex role I had held up to that time. I had little direct power and a great deal of responsibility. In order to achieve my goals, I had to refine and strengthen my skills in collaboration, persuasion, and team building. In staff positions, most of the people you depend on to carry out actions and meet objectives don't work for you. Intimidation and table pounding don't work.

This proactive approach to risk-taking and volunteering established my credibility in the organization. I was appointed to the national utilization management policy board and to the national quality improvement committee. I led projects on improving the quality of claims administration by establishing a continuous quality improvement approach to claims management. I became the business leader for Prudential's start-up mental health managed care business unit until it was turned over to a psychiatrist business leader. The biggest growth opportunity I was given was to be the business leader in charge of improving the existing mainframe computer-based utilization management system while developing a completely new application using an integrated approach with all other managed care computer systems. Each one of these assignments allowed me to work with other business leaders in Prudential, glean best practices, locate new mentors, and test my skills. The lesson learned here is that it is important to demonstrate flexibility and a willingness to work in areas that are not directly related to clinical issues.

In October 1993, I became Executive Director of PruCare Operations in New York, New Jersey, and Connecticut. This was a planned action on my part. Approximately 3 years earlier, I had let my boss and her replacement know that for my next career move, I wanted a job leading a large multifunctional operational unit. I asked what I needed to do to achieve this. Both bosses suggested skills I should acquire, interactive training opportunities and smaller operational assignments I should consider to add to my experience. It is important to discuss career goals with associates and ask for frank feedback as to how to obtain those goals. People are not mind-readers. For instance, I was quite open about my willingness to move for the right opportunity.

That opportunity came unexpectedly in 1998 when Prudential Healthcare was purchased by Aetna US Healthcare. I was given the chance to lead part of the transition—particularly the integration of the data warehouse and the clinical quality and medical cost data analysis teams into the structure of USQA, the analytical arm of Aetna. While helping 367 individuals locate their 'landing' zone within the business units of Aetna, I learned entirely new areas of the business and sharpened my political skills to locate and use leverage to assist staff find positions in or to smooth their exit out of the company. During the transition I also had to deal with five separate changes of management in eight months. Eventually I was given the position of leading the regional analytical teams for USQA. Data and its effective use became the center of my work universe.

One area of skill everyone in medicine today must possess is how to use and analyze data—both clinical and financial. At the moment, Excel proficiency is critical. Physician managers should know how to do pivot tables, the basics of medical coding (service level and diagnosis level), how to read a profit and loss report, balance sheet and how to develop a business budget. These are vital skills that are not learned in medical school.

While advanced degrees can be helpful, it is not the only way to acquire specific business skills. There are inexpensive local community college courses offered on nights and weekends. The American Association of Community Colleges (www.aacc.nche.edu) provides links to these schools.

After managing the analytical teams for USQA, the reorganization of Aetna (and USQA) led to another transition opportunity in 2001. I was given two options:

take a 'regular' medical management role or lead the transition of my teams into the new business structure with a severance package. I opted for the latter. This was not long after September 11th and I wanted to do something different.

With the help of an old friend, I found "different". I had been reading and hearing about managed Medicaid and a new product called Medicare Advantage. A failed experiment in the mid 90's in Medicaid at Prudential had given me a healthy regard for the complexities of taking care of the poorest of the poor. Visiting with pioneers in this line of business convinced me it would be very different. I joined AmeriChoice, attracted by the sharp vision of the leadership team and the fact that I would need to acquire a whole new set of skills for the alternative world of government programs. I led the medical management team of care managers, case managers and utilization review professionals working in the New York and New Jersey markets.

My experience highlights the fact that as a medical manager one needs to constantly keep up with all the latest trends in the world of healthcare. That requires using a mix of sources—newspapers (the Wall Street Journal is the best for the business impact point of view), email alerts from industry watchers (Modern Healthcare is one great source), association bulletins (AMA News is tops even for non-members). Anyone seeking an administrative role in healthcare should invest in various subscriptions to maintain their edge.

For me, my professional landscape continued to change. UnitedHealthcare purchased AmeriChoice in 2005. With the integration into UHC, I moved onto the national team, utilizing my past medical cost analysis and data processing skills to help lead the installation of claim editing software and supporting the implementation of a new claims system for the Medicaid products. I continued to work on medical cost and other special projects while AmeriChoice went through multiple re-alignments until 2008 when I turned down the opportunity to return to a "regular" medical management role and took another severance package starting the search again for something different.

While sitting in the sun in Ridgewood an old friend walked up and asked if I knew anyone with Medicaid experience in managed care looking for a job. I answered, "Depending on what the job is, I may be; I want something different." He told me about a HOSPITAL owned managed care company in New York City seeking a Medical Director to help start a branch in New Jersey. It was different from my past experience: provider owned and managed and a start-up. I joined the organization in 2008, now working in both New Jersey and New York as Healthfirst expands into new Medicare, SNP, managed long term care and health home lines of business.

Final Words of Wisdom

It is not always easy to be a leader, but the role can be extremely reward-ing. Moreover, physician leaders who are able to straddle both the clinical and business sides of medicine possess skills that are truly unique. As one of my greatest mentors, Ron C., a senior operational leader said, "Deborah, remem-ber you (medical directors) have turf that no one else can step into, but every-one in this (healthcare) organization has turf you CAN step into. Your turf is nearly infinite, so be very careful not to 'blank' it up without a plan of entrance (and exit)". Because he was a profane Texan, I can't do justice to how he actu-ally worded it. Dialogue right out of a Larry McMurtry novel.

For physician executives, accountability stops with you. As an administrator, that means your desk, your email, your signature (which is now digital), your attestation. If you are the top clinical leader in your organization and a medi-cal decision is needed, there is no other place or person to delegate the task. Even when the decision concerns some operational aspect of your business, if that operation involves patient care, you will likely be involved. What makes this so rewarding is the fact that you can have great influence over the even-tual decision and steps taken for the good of the organization while serving patient care needs.

If you are interested in leadership in medicine, the opportunities are out there for women (and men) with many pathways for entrance. Look for open-ings at the practice level, the department level, the health system level, the state and federal government in additional to managed care companies and insurers.

In addition to acquiring hard skills, I would advise learning to be an extrovert. Most physicians test as introverts on the Myers-Briggs personality test. Take the test, learn about your "type" and learn how to move out of type to con-nect with people, including gaining experience in public speaking (said to be the most dreaded voluntary activity in the world). Toastmasters International (www.toastmasters.org) is an international leader in communication and lead-ership development. There are chapters in every part of America. Over the years many of my "new" recruits to administration have joined and gained the skills needed to stand out in a crowd.

Even if you are just recently out of medical school and residency, consider some aspect of administration as a future option—whether you think you might want to be a senior medical leader or not. Volunteer. Credentialing, chart review, audit/accreditation preparation, practice management tasks, electronic medical record implementation, clinical guideline development provide excellent experience (even if unpaid) and more importantly, networking opportunities. In my experience, most organizations will appreciate your offer to help. They are especially interested in younger women physicians who are usually "too busy" to do such work or worry their offer would be rejected.

If you are worried about initial rejection, network with other leaders in the organization to obtain advice on how to gain "entrance". Volunteering as a first step is especially important if you are a minority or represent a distinct cultural group. Look to your cultural peers for help. In the populated northeast there are active associations such as the Korean-American Physician Association, which have and know how to use political leverage to aide their peers in obtaining the proverbial "seat-at-the-table".

Networking is key to discovering options open in medical management. Find those you hope to emulate and simply ask: "How did you get your job? Why do you like it? What would you change if you could? How can I get a job like yours?" In most cases, you will find people willing to provide guidance and share their expertise. Not only will information pour out, but the person you've asked will likely remember you!

Impact of 2014

So where are the opportunities today? One date sums it up: 2014. That's the date when most of the provisions in the Affordable Care Act will be implemented (assuming the mandate is not found unconstitutional and the entire legislation overturned). I recommend reading Edward Tenner's 1996 *Why Things Bite Back; Technology and the Revenge of Unintended Consequences.* Consider what are the unintended consequences you can anticipate given the proposed changes and act upon those opportunities to your advantage.

ObamaCare will open a flood of health care resources to manage in 2014. Health systems will need to manage the unruly mix of physicians and other professional service providers they have placed or plan to place under a single structure. Many systems still use a modified "share-of-billings" or payment-for-each-service method to reimburse the professionals—especially the specialists. To get ready, in 2012, these same health systems are developing detailed, realistic, financial plans. They know the rate of the rise of reimbursement from all payer sources is dropping and may go negative in the next few years. They know their current "mousetrap" won't be effective in the future, but they are not sure what will work. They are looking for people who can help figure it out.

The Accountable Care Organization (ACO) is the government's current answer to what should work. However, taking an ACO from concept to reality will require leveraging medical leadership to manage an evolution/revolution in medical practice with many hours of toil (and trouble).

An ACO is basically an "insured" population in disguise. You are given a "risk adjusted" revenue stream for each attributed member (think premium), you are asked to manage all aspects of the care with a selected panel of physicians and providers (think managed care network), you are expected to ensure access and quality of care (think regulatory requirements) while placing dollars at risk for your administrative costs and devising ways to incentivize doctors financially to provide the right care (think utilization management) within a budget.

Recently published results on the early ACO pilots (funded by CMS) showed little success to tout to the press. There is no end of opportunity for physicians to enter some type or level of leadership position in organizations struggling to find a path to success.

I believe ObamaCare could be renamed the "full employment act for physician leaders". Regardless of the Supreme court's action, the American system of healthcare will change profoundly in the near term. The drive for improved outcomes and reduced cost will create many "broken" processes that will require rethinking the provision of health care in ways you, your peers, and administrators have never considered.

Making it Work

I firmly believe that you cannot have it all. You will have to pick and choose and plan your career carefully in order to create a balance between work and the rest of your life. Make a list of what is essential to you (e.g. marriage, having children, time for specific avocations, etc)

This is especially important for women. Many of my classmates from the 70's found they had waited too long to have children. We did not know about the "senile" eggs of a 30 year old and the stress-induced infertility seen in professional women. Today young women have that knowledge; use this information in your life plan calculation.

We are lucky in other ways as women in medicine. First, we are exposed to many potential, highly educated mates. Data suggests a high probability of finding a life partner among them. Second, we will have a predictable income stream (even after paying off the loans) for life. There will be both full-time and part-time opportunities for clinical and administrative work.

Third, whether you marry a medical colleague or not, you will likely be a two-income family. This means you can afford to live in a neighborhood with great schools or pay private tuition even if you enter a primary care practice as your career starting point. Many medical practices today are willing to accommodate families of two professionals knowing how many physicians are now linked to a working spouse/significant other.

Personally, I have had a housekeeper from the year my husband and I set up our household and later a nanny AND a housekeeper. Don't expect either of you to change the linens or do the toilets (unless that is how you relax).

Working in medical administration can allow for as much if not more flexibility than straight clinical practice. Most positions require regular work hours (no swing shifts) and you have holidays and liberal vacation time allotments. You can (with a bit of planning) go to school meetings, athletic events and take the kids on the usual calendar of vacations. Some regional or national positions require travel, but once again, you can make it work. Most businesses work very hard to accommodate and retain high potential/high cost executive women. So learn about the benefits offered and use them.

In terms of management roles, those physicians trained in primary care specialties generally have an advantage—at least in managed care organizations. Pediatricians, Internists and Family Practitioners are the most versatile and sought after for leadership positions. As the demographics in the US change, those trained in Geriatrics will find growing opportunities, so if you are already trained in adult medicine, consider a fellowship if you believe you eventually want to become an administrator.

One of the questions I am often asked is whether a physician leader needs to continue direct clinical practice. Realistically, once you begin working more than 20 hours a week in administration, you are less available to your patients—especially if you are in primary care. Who wants to hear their doctor is out 50 percent of the time when they call for help?

Personally, I still consider myself to be in clinical practice in the sense that as an administrator I review the care of patients both retrospectively and prospectively many times each and every day. The oversight dictated by regulators and the expectations of the public require applying a critical eye toward appropriateness and quality. In my administrative role, I often have to answer this question: "With the information presented, is the care clinically effective and in the best interests of the patient?" This requires my keeping up with advances in medicine and connecting with practicing physicians.

Finally, be proud of being a physician leader. The role is vital to a successful healthcare business. There is no reason to be defensive when discussing what you do. As a medical manager, you enable people to get the care they need. By using the considerable resources of your organization, you create paths for the clinical physicians and other health care providers to follow in order to provide effective care. Many changes are on the horizon and health care resources are finite. It will take physician leaders to make it all work. Join us on the "other" side. If you do, I promise you will never be bored.

CHAPTER SEVENTEEN

Behind Every Good Woman – Good Mentors

by Traci Ferguson, MD

My mother, a nursing assistant, exposed me early to the healthcare profession. When I had a day off from elementary school, she would bring me to work and I would pass out graham crackers and juice to the nursing home residents. As the first physician in my family, my decision to become a doctor was not solidified until I was almost twelve years old. While in middle school, I got my first job babysitting for Peggy Sugar, a semi-retired nurse. After almost twenty years as a registered nurse Mrs. Sugar decided to quit her job and stay at home with her son. One day I shared my thoughts for a future career in medical technology. Aware of my recent acceptance into the International Baccalaureate program, she asked why I didn't want to be a doctor. She told me that even at my age, I was smarter than some of physicians she knew and said that I should become a doctor. That did it for me! From that moment on becoming a doctor became my goal.

When I tell people about the origins of my career decision, they are uniformly amazed at how that one simple statement changed the course of my life. That episode in time illustrates the power of positive belief. Mrs. Sugar believed that I could become a doctor. As a result of her belief in me, I believed that I could achieve that goal and so much more. My subsequent undergraduate and medical school choices of Georgetown University and Johns Hopkins University School of Medicine, respectively, were firmly grounded in the belief that I could achieve great things if I aligned my thoughts and actions with my desired end. This is why it is so important to carefully choose mentors who want the best for you, who want you to succeed, who believe that you can achieve and encourage you to dream big.

To better foster a relationship between medical students and faculty, all medical students at Hopkins were assigned an advisor. The four-year advisor program encouraged an active exchange between student and faculty. My advisor and mentor was Dr. Fred Brancati, an internist with a strong research interest. While still a medical student I worked on his clinical trial as part of the Diabetes Prevention Program. I really enjoyed interviewing and following patients during their visits. My desire for bedside interaction with patients was one of the reasons I chose to pursue a residency in internal medicine. My work with Dr. Brancati allowed me to interact with other members of the general internal medicine faculty including Dr. Lisa Cooper who became my role model and second mentor. Her research on racial disparities within healthcare and her work to bring greater attention to the needs of women and minorities at Hopkins inspired me to always strive to do more.

I initially contemplated fellowship training in general internal medicine, which included completion of a Masters degree in Public Health. However, the paucity of women in tenured positions in academic medicine in the mid-1990s made me reevaluate my initial decision to enter academic medicine early in my career. Another less spoken reason was the lack of timely and successful advancement of purely clinical physicians in academia during that time. The research track was well established. but the clinical track was largely unchartered. I clearly saw the gender disparity between the advancement of men and women in academic medicine. Not to say that such disparity in position and pay did not also exist outside of academics. However, in hospital medicine I saw greater equality and growth potential. I also could capitalize on the flexibility and transferability of skills if I ever chose to return to academic medicine. At that phase in my life, I turned to colleagues and other professionals in the field to help navigate my transition from residency to clinical practice. After talking with fellow female residents in medicine and other primary care specialties, about thirty percent of my third year class of internal medicine residents decided to enter general practice and not sub-specialize which was a significant break from the Hopkins tradition. I chose to go into hospital medicine because of work life balance. With a more predictable schedule I would have more time for my future family, which came five years later with the birth of my first child.

During my tenure in hospital medicine I continued to explore my interest in academics by teaching medical students and working with administration on quality improvement projects. I collaborated with case management and other hospital ancillary departments to ensure timely patient disposition and transitions of care. This experience exposed me to the world of administrative medicine. As medical director of a hospital medicine program I was responsible for tracking and reporting the physicians' adherence to core quality measures and developed a pay for performance program to achieve one hundred percent compliance with these metrics.

With over eleven years of practicing medicine at the bedside, I acquired first-hand experience in caring for a forgotten portion of society, the uninsured and underinsured. I observed numerous people turning to the emergency room as their last, and often their only resort for healthcare. Many individuals who had state-sponsored health plans still frequented the emergency department. Their assigned physicians were often too busy with routine office visits to squeeze in urgent same-day appointments. All too often, I witnessed the difficulties patients experience in navigating through a complex system like government-sponsored healthcare. I would often personally call to schedule follow-up appointments for patients before they left the hospital, especially if I knew the task would be onerous. When a young woman finally confessed to me "it's hard to be on Medicaid because no one wants to take your insurance," I realized I needed to do more.

Coinciding with my desire to address the increasing social demands on my patients, I had reached a point in my career where I needed to recalibrate the work-life balance. After returning to work following the birth of my second child, the reality of fourteen-hour shifts began to take its toil. So I turned to physician executive recruiter, Dr. Deborah Shlian. Dr. Shlian possessed an invaluable breath of experience and perspective given her expansive background in managed care. She helped me realize that all of my prior experience managing physicians' behavior and practice patterns could easily translate into the arena of managed care. Armed with this timely advice, I welcomed the opportunity to join WellCare Health Plans, Inc. as a medical director of utilization and care management.

I transitioned from clinical practice to managed care because I wanted to focus on improving access to quality care for an entire population, and not just for individuals. Although I currently work full-time as a managed care medical director I continue to work as a hospital-based physician some weekends a month so I can still help the most vulnerable individuals negotiate the healthcare system. I believe that my continued practice of clinical medicine gives me increased credibility when discussing care management issues with providers. I am also able to voice member, provider and hospital concerns when it comes to my company's managed care policies. In my dual role as practicing physician and health plan administrator, I can make decisions that reflect my own high standards of care. I take immense pride in knowing that countless members and providers benefit from my accumulated clinical experience.

People, especially other physicians, often ask me how I entered administrative medicine. After I describe the events of my journey, they come to realize the importance of knowing and connecting with the right people at the right time. This statement is certainly true of my relationship with Dr. Vincent Kunz, my first supervisor at WellCare. As a general surgeon who had spent over seventeen years in practice before assuming the role as medical director over a multi-specialty group, he openly admitted that he entered administrative medicine late in his career. He became an ideal mentor for me because he freely provided me with advice and encouragement and took it upon himself to expose me to all aspects of managed care. He had an open-door policy and urged me to attend various committees and interdepartmental meetings to expand my knowledge base.

I believe the best mentors are the people who do not see the mentee's ambition as a threat to their own professional success. I have found the best advisors among my colleagues who are well anchored in their career or on the tail end of their career. They do not have anything to fear from my questioning and frequently welcome the opportunity to cultivate my interest. During one of our weekly one-on-one sessions, Dr. Kunz advised me to obtain an advanced management degree since I was early in my career in administrative medicine. Never one to second guess sage advice, I began researching executive MBA programs. As I often do, I consulted my husband who wholeheartedly agreed that now was the time to pursue my MBA. Being in a very business minded environment, I knew an MBA would be more easily recognized and accepted than other advanced management degrees.

I sought to find the best program that would provide an expansive breadth of knowledge and the flexibility I needed with two small children at home. I chose Howard University's online Executive MBA program to achieve my professional goal of becoming an effective physician leader while allowing me to continue in my current position without disruption in my administrative responsibilities. During a mock interview session with my medical school mentor, I told him that my goal in life is "to run something big." Although that statement shocked him and even caught me off guard for a moment, it appears fitting when I look at my career trajectory. I graduated with honors from a top ranked medical school, completed my internal medicine residency training at a world-renowned medical institution, and accumulated over six years of managerial experience leading up my decision to pursue an advanced management degree at Howard University.

With an MBA on the horizon, I envision my entrance into senior management in the next five to ten years. Increased advancement opportunities are now available for female physician executives both in the private and academic sectors. Academic medicine has made significant strides over the past ten years in solidifying the succession process of a number of well-deserving women who are now full professors, department chairs and hospital executives. I am proud to say that one of my medical school mentors, Dr. Cooper, who was an assistant professor some ten years ago is now a full professor and the recipient of the prestigious "genius award"—the MacArthur Fellowship—for her groundbreaking work on health disparities. Both academic institutions and private healthcare companies now realize the imperative to address the needs of the female physician executive. For me, family and personal commitments ultimately weigh heavy on my career choices. Many of my female colleagues agree that maintaining flexibility in their schedule to attend school and professional conferences, fair remuneration for their skills and talent, and timely promotions are important considerations for job selection and loyalty.

With the rising costs of healthcare and increasing demands on our human and financial capital, physicians across all sectors face ever-changing priorities to deliver high quality, efficient and effective care for all stakeholders involved. My transition from purely clinical practice to administrative medicine was a natural progression for me. I witnessed the challenges of a hospital system as it realigned physician incentives to reflect quality performance and patient outcomes. Now working in a managed care organization I see a similar paradigm shift linking fiscal growth to quality measures. I knew that I needed to expand my business acumen to be a successful physician executive in the healthcare industry. The business strategies and skills that I will learn in the executive MBA program will allow me to critically analyze current business processes to identify and eliminate areas of excess and waste, and develop a more efficient work flow of evidence-based standards in care delivery.

My journey as a physician executive is just beginning. One of the keys to my early entrance into administrative medicine is finding the right mentor at the right time. In my life and career, I found that mentors are for a time and come in many different forms. Little did I realize that one conversation with a semi-retired nurse at the age of twelve would translate into a blossoming career in medicine and now as a physician executive. The full affect of an individual's influence on your life is usually not evident until many years later. Additionally, the far-reaching effects of personal decisions made years and decades ago often meld together seamlessly to form your current career trajectory.

I receive the most of my relationship with my mentors when I fully commit myself to achieving my desired goal. My mentors provide me the specific bar or target to reach and in turn, I lay the foundation and cultivate my actions to attain that goal and beyond. Like any journey, my list of mentors is unique and eclectic, from semi-retired nurse—my first official employer at the age of twelve, my childhood friend's father, my undergraduate work-study employer, my medical school advisor and mentors, my physician executive recruiter, and without question, my husband, Rhadi Ferguson PhD. My husband has been my constant supporter and personal mentor. His keen insight and entrepreneurial spirit adds a refreshing vantage point when making these life-changing decisions. I credit his selflessness in helping me make choices that are good for both my career and for our family.

CHAPTER EIGHTEEN

Medicine and Leadership: An Unplanned Journey

by Eugenie Komives, MD

I was born with multiple vascular anomalies that led the doctors to tell my parents I might not survive to leave the hospital after birth. Obviously, I did.... But I spent more time in hospitals and doctor offices by the time I graduated from high school than most folks probably do in a lifetime. I do not remember much about any of those experiences except that I grew up feeling different from my classmates and tried to hide my "different-ness" much of the time.

I was not able to participate in physical education and that gave me more time for academic classes in which I always excelled and mostly found pretty easy. I also played the flute and for a while thought I'd be a flautist when I grew up. That changed when I went off to a band camp at UW Madison and was 30th chair out of 60 flute players. I realized I'd likely end up a high school band director if I continued to focus only on music as a career. Nothing against band directors, but I could not envision a life dealing with surly teenagers.

My best friend's father was a radiation oncologist and cancer researcher, and after a brief period of thinking about veterinary medicine (I was allergic to cats!) I entertained biochemistry and research. After graduating as valedictorian of my high school, I started at UW Madison to study chemistry and biology.

My father was a small business consultant (his focus was the study of the psychology of entrepreneurs) and my mother was a frustrated math and science major who did her masters degree in home economics because in her day "if you went to graduate school in science or math, you would never marry". She drilled into her daughters the importance of having our own careers (but did make sure we also knew how to type!) Both of my parents were very demanding of their daughters' education and expected that we would be straight "A" students. It was never said that we could not accomplish something because of our gender.

None of my family members was a physician, however. My parents were not wealthy. My mom made all our clothes. I remember the first time she let us buy a pair of Levi's late in high school – it was such a splurge. However, my parents scrimped and saved so that we were all able to go to college.

While in college, I was often asked why I was not a "pre-med", since I excelled in science and math there as well. It was just not on my radar screen. However, I had the misfortune of suffering a retroperitoneal hemorrhage (related to my vascular birth defects) while on a family vacation in Quebec, Canada. I was left in horrible pain and during that hospitalization, I clearly remember having some "interesting" physicians. One was a neurologist who barely spoke to me, and inflicted pain on every visit (and was seemingly unconcerned about this.) The other was a hematologist (the first woman I ever had as a physician!) who was caring, kind, and took the time to talk with me about what was happening. I remember thinking at the time that the world needed more physicians like her, and fewer like him, and that maybe I should be one of the empathetic ones.

I returned to Wisconsin, and after a long recovery, got back on my feet and continued my junior year of college. Though I did not immediately change career paths, after a stint in a research lab, I realized that I needed more people around me to be happy. That was the point when I realized that I should go to medical school. Fortunately, my courses prepared me well so I was able to graduate on time with my classmates. I applied to several medical schools. Some had me interview with only men, some of whom were less than supportive of filling medical schools with women. Others clearly made an effort to demonstrate that women were welcome, using women faculty as interviewers. At that time (1980), women comprised roughly 25 percent of medical students in the US.

My younger sister was enrolled at MIT for college, and encouraged (read: FORCED) me to apply to Harvard Medical School. Much to my surprise I was accepted. We planned to live together while she was still there, and so I moved to Boston (I had never lived in a true city.) I met my future husband on my first day of medical school. We began dating a few months later, and moved in together after completing our first year of med school. He is a wonderful, supportive, grounded fellow and I love him as much now as I did when we first met. Once asked what the secret to a long relationship with a "Komives" woman was, he remarked (after a moment's thought), "If she says she's going to do something, get out of the way." I think that response typifies the sort of support he provides – he's there when I need him (which I often do), but does not get in the way.

My husband had taken a year off from medical school to do some research, so while waiting for him to graduate, I did a one-year internship in internal medicine at Beth Israel in Boston. I was never so miserable as I watched way too many young people die. I felt my inability to "fix" them was a failing on my part.

Originally I had planned to do a residency in Ob-Gyn once my husband finished medical school. However, he had done a 1-month clerkship in Family Medicine in rural Maine, and reminded me that Family Medicine had once been my goal. The support for primary care at Harvard at the time was minimal to none so I'd given up the idea. However, after some thought and reading, I decided my husband was a very wise man, and I applied for Family Medicine residencies, while he applied in Pathology.

We matched together at Duke, where the director of the Family Medicine residency was a woman who I will always think of as one of my main mentors. She was strong, ethical, patient oriented, tough, and kind. She was also a wife (of another family physician), and a parent. She believed that women could "do it all" if we just put our minds to it. While in residency, I worked with many other wise, wonderful women as residents and faculty. Many of them remain close friends and colleagues today.

I also learned that behaviors that were acceptable from male residents were frequently not tolerated from the women. For example, while men could "tell" staff what they needed, we were expected to politely ask, or we would be labeled as "difficult" or "bitchy". While I believe this gender differentiation is unfair and unreasonable, perhaps medicine would be better served if ALL providers had to politely ask for what we needed in the care of our patients. Needless to say, I was pragmatic enough to temper my "bull in a china shop" attitude and work collaboratively with my colleagues.

After finishing my residency, I contemplated a career in public health. My husband still had several years more of residency and research before he would be ready to settle on a job. Realizing that for at least a while I really just wanted to be a primary care physician, I finally took a position with Kaiser Permanente in Durham for what I assumed would be a few years stint before we would both move on. Little did I know that the Kaiser Permanente pre-paid integrated model was the perfect clinical fit for me. I truly believed then, as I do now, that we do best for our patients when we provide them with ALL of the health care they need, and yet ONLY the health care that they will benefit from, using the evidence as well as the art, to guide our decisions.

I had never planned a career in management, but when the chief of Family Medicine role became available, I asked to take that on. I think this was born of my desire to "fix things", and a need to feel like I had some influence on how care was delivered. Despite the fact that our area medical director, probably rightfully, felt I was not ready for the role (only 3 years into my career as practicing physician), he let me assume the position on condition that I agree to mentor with one of our senior female physician leaders. Though she and I were as different as night and day, she took her responsibility seriously, providing me timely and helpful advice as I moved into the management role.

Kaiser also had a management training program that taught me the basics of management (e.g., how to run a meeting, how to influence others, the difference between leadership and management, how to provide performance evaluations and have "difficult" conversations.) It also gave me the opportunity to meet other physician leaders, including many women. After only 2 years, I applied for an associate medical director position (a 70 percent administrative role). I was so excited and proud that our executive medical director had the confidence to offer me the job. However, immediately after our first "senior" staff meeting during which I had remained silent, trying to take it all in and figure out my role, he criticized my lack of participation. "I did not hire you to sit there quietly," he said. "I want to hear your thoughts and opinions as a part of this team. They are critical to me, and to our success." This was a real eye-opener. I have since learned that this was the type of leader I need to seek out. I need to be comfortable to be me – to share what I'm thinking and my opinions – openly and without concern, in order to be both satisfied in my role and also to be the best leader I can in my organization.

Unfortunately, unlike other parts of the country where Kaiser Permanente is a stable force in the market (e.g. California), that was not the case in the North Carolina market. Prepaid healthcare in a restricted network was a foreign concept in our market, and we attracted "adverse risk" from an underwriting perspective, while our largest client (the NC State Health Plan) charged us an extra fee because our members were slightly younger than the average (though I believe we took on every hemophiliac in their member population, for example.) Ultimately, we were simply too expensive for our parent company in California to continue to support, so they made a decision to divest themselves of the North Carolina market. (For a more detailed analysis of this, see Daniel P. Gitterman et al; "The Rise and Fall of a Kaiser Permanente Expansion Region", The Millbank Quarterly, 81:4, 2003 (567-601).)

After an 11-year run with Kaiser, and a 10 month period back in full time clinical practice, the remaining physician group went out of business. Luckily, just in time, I was offered a position with Blue Cross and Blue Shield of North Carolina by the same physician who had hired me out of residency for Kaiser. I had a wonderful opportunity to work with an outspoken, strong, open minded man who took over the leadership of our State Health Plan, and worked himself (and the rest of us) as hard as possible to make changes needed to bring it back to fiscal solvency. He trusted my judgment in all things clinical, and I learned a tremendous amount from him about the finances and business of running a health plan.

When he retired, I took a position as a senior medical director, and soon vice president, managing BCBSNC's healthcare quality programs. In that role, I have had to deliver many difficult messages to my fellow physicians, all in the interest of improving the quality, and the evidence-base, of care delivered to our members, their patients. I have spent countless hours meeting with representatives of the medical society, various specialty academies, hospital leaders, and others, to help them understand how we can better partner together to achieve our shared vision of improved healthcare in North Carolina.

After almost 12 years working in the insurance world, I can look back at what I've accomplished and see that being a physician leader allowed me to make just as important contributions to the care of patients as I had as a clinician. For example, my colleagues and I have reinvented payment for primary care physicians in smaller independent practices, focusing on achieving "patient centered medical homes" and rewarding doctors financially according to that effort. We have implemented programs with partner organizations such as the North Carolina Academy of Family Physicians to increase the numbers of medical students going into primary care in the state. We have stimulated improvement in the care patients receive during hospitalization as well as at the time of discharge. We have reduced the number of patients who inappropriately undergo imaging procedures and some surgical procedures. I am proud of all of these accomplishments, but I am most proud of the fact that we did this while creating collaborative and friendly working relationship with physicians across the state who share our goals of improving care for patients. In honor of that collaboration, I have been awarded a "President's Award" from the NCAFP, and have been asked to take over the leadership of our North Carolina Medical Society Foundation's Leadership Scholars Program, which develops physician leaders for North Carolina. The use of "we" above is very intentional – I have had a wonderful team of nurses and other staff who have taken my crazy ideas and made them reality through their hard work and commitment to our goals.

All that said, I do miss the care of patients, and had always envisioned returning to the clinical world. That opportunity recently came when a practice affiliated with Duke Primary Care in my small town decided to add another physician. I am honored to be joining the group, practicing with physicians I have known for many years including a close colleague from Kaiser Permanente. Though this feels like another big "leap" and no doubt will be a difficult transition, these doctors are committed to helping me be successful. My part time clinical role will also create a bit of space in my life to take on different leadership roles in the future within the physician community in North Carolina.

My professional success has not come without a price. My husband and I adopted twin infant girls from Vietnam in 1996, who at one time thought their mommy lived in California (due to travel for Kaiser Permanente work.) Fortunately, my husband and I have been able to share the family duties roughly 50-50. I have missed many soccer games, track meets, cross country meets, and parent-teacher conferences, but so has my husband – and one of us has been at almost all of them. That said, I think my now 15 year-old daughters have come to understand that in terms of career options, being a girl is no different than being a boy. They understand that sometimes we must work harder than we want to, and that we all make choices and need to be accountable for them. I do not think I would have been a better parent if I had stayed at home with my children, though that does not stop me from feeling guilty when I talk with moms that made different decisions.

Most recently, I have enjoyed the opportunity to mentor other younger leaders who are just starting their careers. It is truly exciting to see that there are new, developing leaders who will take what we've put in place, improve it or throw it away, and continue the commitment to improving healthcare that each prior generation has fostered.

It should be clear from my story that my career has been less than intentional. I have wandered into many roles that have been interesting and exciting, without ever having had a "plan" or what felt like true "ambition". I did not set my sights on being a leader in a medical practice or in a health plan. However, I did take advantage of opportunities as they came along, and at my core have followed my desire to serve and to lead.

My advice to other women physician leaders is to do your best to keep some balance in your life. Too often, women who attempt to do it all have a difficult time asking for help. We don't allot enough time to take care of ourselves which includes spending time with our family and friends. It is too easy to let the career take control of our lives, at the risk of losing other things of greater value in the long run. Let's collectively seek balance not just for us but for our husbands, sons, and daughters, by insisting on the changes needed in our workplaces to assure that they will be sustainable into the future.

CHAPTER NINETEEN

Finding the Right Niche

by Elaine E. Batchlor, MD, MPH

I knew from a young age that I wanted to be a doctor and my career in medicine and management has been shaped by the ideas I developed about medicine when I was first attracted to it. As I child, I transported myself through books and at some time during my childhood I read a novel by Taylor Caldwell, called *Dear and Glorious Physician*. This novel portrayed the life of a physician in ancient times as one devoted to healing, expanding knowledge, promoting public health and battling socioeconomic causes of disease and disability. Although it may appear that a career in medical management is a far cry from being a physician in ancient Rome, the characterization of medicine brought to life in *Dear and Glorious Physician* inspired me and formed a lasting framework for my subsequent education and career. Even today. as a mature physician executive, this portrayal fits my view of who I am and what I do.

I studied the history, development, and social aspects of medicine and health care as an undergraduate and later as a graduate student in public health. I developed a career in medical management in order to actively participate in shaping the ongoing evolution of medicine and health care delivery.

Although I understand how I got where I am today, and it fits and satisfies me, I wouldn't say that I planned it. I started out in medicine like most other students, with a vague notion of a specialty I would pursue and with the confidence that a job would await me at the end of my training. I decided to be an internist because I was attracted to the emphasis placed on intellectual rumination and the collegiality of the internists with whom I clerked. After completing a residency in internal medicine, I signed on for a fellowship in rheumatology. During my residency and fellowship, I traversed ground that placed me on the path to medical management.

I spent the five years of my residency and fellowship at a county hospital affiliated with UCLA. It was a strong training program but a typical county hospital. I gained a firsthand view of the problems that the poor experience in attempting to access medical care. I also experienced the frustration of a physician attempting to provide care within the constraints of a suboptimal system. I saw ways in which the system could be changed to better serve its mission of caring for the poor. At some point, I was struck by the thought that I might accomplish more to help my patients by attempting to reshape the system than by caring for them one by one.

I was fortunate to have a rheumatology program director who shared a broad view of the mission of medicine. He guided me toward working on a health services research project with colleagues at UCLA's Schools of Medicine and Public Health. During the research year of my fellowship, I worked on a project designed to test the impact of teaching rheumatoid arthritis patients to participate in making medical decisions with their doctors. The year following my fellowship, I joined the faculty at UCLA Medical School to continue work on the project. My agreement with the Division of Rheumatology was that I would begin to build a career doing health services research in rheumatology. And, I would strengthen my training for such a career by completing a master's level program at UCLA's School of Public Health.

At this point, I made a somewhat uninformed but conscious choice that furthered my progress toward a career in medical management. I enrolled in a health services MPH program rather than in an epidemiology program. Epidemiology would have been more valuable training for a research career, but health services was what appealed to me. Health Services focused on themes that excited me—the history of medicine, the evolution of health care financing and organization, the sociopolitical forces influencing health care policy, and the challenge of providing care for poor and underserved communities. I was surprised that I enjoyed being a student again; learning new things invigorated me. I was also stimulated by the ideas and experiences of my fellow students, predominantly other professionals who shared similar interests.

After I completed my master's degree in public health, I realized that I didn't want to be an academician. The pace of discovery and impact on health care proceeds slowly in research; I just wasn't patient enough to find it fulfilling. I also found it too solitary a pursuit, with a lot of time devoted to writing papers and grants. I wanted a job where I could more directly affect the health care that people receive and where I would accomplish my goals by working closely with other people.

I thought about a career in public health and enrolled in a residency in preventive medicine, while remaining on the medical school faculty. I visited physicians who were public health officers to learn about their jobs. I took the state exam for public health officers and waited for a letter announcing a job opening.

While I was waiting, I received a call from a friend in my preventive medicine residency. She asked whether I would be interested in a position as a physician administrator in a staff-model HMO. I interviewed with a physician executive, also from UCLA, whom I liked very much. At that point, I had to make a difficult decision. I was torn over whether to abandon an opportunity for an academic career in order to pursue a new, uncertain path. I felt comfortable in knowing what was expected of me as an academician. I didn't know what a career in medical management would bring.

I finally decided to take the risk. I knew that it was time to make a change, and I believed that my future boss would support my development and learning. Luckily, I was right on both accounts. I accepted a position as chief of staff for a multispecialty ambulatory health care center that was part of a staff model health plan. This position entailed managing physicians, other health care professionals, support staff, and the operations of a busy outpatient clinic.

This job turned out to be a wonderful opportunity to discover and develop management and leadership skills and to work on improving health care operations. I learned the value of teamwork and of continuous quality improvement. An engaged and empowered staff began to make progress on long-standing challenges, such as ensuring medical records availability, reducing office wait times, and managing appointment scheduling. I also learned how to work effectively with practicing physicians, helping them understand and embrace the importance of customer service and cost-effective clinical practice. I enjoyed the opportunities for continuous learning and working on activities as diverse as capital budgeting, architectural plans for new building, and clinical practice. I was fortunate to have a boss who threw challenges at me, supported me in my efforts to meet them, and gave me credit and visibility for my successes.

My successes as a manager led to broader responsibilities over time. Eventually, I became a service area medical director responsible for four ambulatory centers and participated in the opening of a new center. After two years with this health plan, I accepted a position as medical director for a network-model HMO. I viewed this as an opportunity to learn about a different type of delivery system and to continue to broaden the scope of my responsibilities.

This transition was easier than the transition from academia because I knew I was on the right path. I continued to work as a health plan medical director for six more years, taking on larger roles, before making another significant transition. After working as a medical director for three health plans, the CEO of a statewide health care foundation asked me to go to work for him as a program officer focusing on health care system issues. Because I wasn't convinced that I would enjoy working in a not-for-profit organization, outside the mainstream of the health care system, and the position required my moving to a different city, I didn't immediately accept. Only after several months of reflection, did I finally decide to give it a try. It turned out that I liked my job at the foundation. During the five years I worked there I was able to step back from the day-to-day management of a health care organization and reflect on how the system and its parts could improve. I collaborated with academics, industry stakeholders and other experts to describe how health care businesses function and how they could work better. I pursued and helped secure funding for innovative ideas to improve various aspects of the system. We addressed issues such as workforce development and deployment, provider payment, quality and performance measurement and the structure and financial performance of health care organizations. I enjoyed working with people who had deep knowledge, broad perspectives and creative ideas about how to improve the quality and efficiency of the health care system. It was challenging and fun to figure out how to use foundation resources to leverage change. It's a whole different perspective when your job is to figure out how to effectively spend money, rather than how to save or make money.

Although I enjoyed the time I spent at the foundation, part of me wanted to jump back into the fray of a health care organization. For the most part, foundations achieve their goals by working through other organizations and people. It's nice to be the person who decides which issues and organizations to fund, but the trade off is giving up the satisfaction of doing the work yourself. And I wasn't entirely ready to give that up. About the same time I began to feel ready for a job change, I was also ready to make major changes in my personal life. I had always had a vague idea that I would like to have a family some day, however, like many professional women, I was more invested in developing my career and was happy to put off having children. Fortunately, I met my husband just in the nick of time. So, at an age when my peers were preparing to send their children off to college, I got married and had two children (twins!).

Starting a family had an impact on my professional life that was both surprising and predictable. I knew that becoming a parent would mean making new accommodations, but I wasn't sure how I would feel about that. After my children were born, I grappled with the need to redefine my priorities and the boundaries of my career. After some soul searching, I realized that I wanted to be available for my children and needed a job that would that would allow me to spend time with them. I reluctantly acknowledged that I was no longer free to pursue whatever opportunity was appealing to me.

My passion for working in a role where I could help improve health care hadn't diminished, however I accepted that I would need to balance career and family obligations. I knew that a job that required significant travel and late office hours wouldn't work for me as the parent of small children. My husband and I also decided that we wanted to live close to our extended families, which required moving back to the city where we had spent most of our professional lives. Fortunately, the right opportunity soon presented itself, and when it did, I recognized it. I jumped at the chance to return to a management role in a regional health care organization and accepted a position as Chief Medical Officer of a regional Medicaid health plan called L.A. Care Health Plan. When I was considering the job, I recall being warned that going to work for a Medicaid health plan might box me into the world of publicly financed health care. After eight years in the same role, I don't believe that is true and I have a very different perspective.

I feel fortunate that my job has not only brought together the strands of my professional interests, but has also worked well for my personal life. I have worked for a not-for-profit, public agency that serves low-income residents of Los Angeles County and strives to improve systems of care for underserved communities. I have loved being part of a mission-driven organization that is about helping our neediest communities. Working for an organization that focuses on a large, but limited geographic region has been a great fit for me. Los Angeles County is large enough to have significant reach and visibility, but small enough to be able to see the impact of the work I do. Being in the leadership of a smaller health plan has given me autonomy, flexibility and nimbleness. Working in the same position for many years has allowed me to develop strong, stable relationships with colleagues inside and outside of my organization. I've been able to set priorities, allocate resources, and collaborate effectively. All of this translates into the ability to innovate and implement ideas and programs that I value.

As this book is about to go to press, I coincidentally find myself on the verge of a significant career change. After eight and a half years as the CMO of L.A.

Care Health Plan, a large, public, Medicaid focused plan, I've accepted an offer to become the CEO of a new hospital.

This hospital is the product of a unique public private partnership between the County of Los Angeles, the University of California and the private board of the new not-for profit Martin Luther King Jr. Community Hospital. The goal of this partnership is to bring a brand new, state of the art hospital to the underserved of South Los Angeles, a community that lost a critical safety net hospital when the previous County-operated Martin Luther King Jr. Medical Center closed in 2007. Scheduled to open in 2014, the hospital will start under the authority of a new private board, with a new facility, start-up and supplemental funding for indigent care from Los Angeles County as well as a commitment from the University of California health system to support provision of physician services and quality of care.

Why am I making this change now? In brief, it feels like the right opportunity and challenge at the right time. The safety net nature of the new hospital is consistent with my passion and the focus of my last eight years as the CMO of an organization working to improve access and quality of care for underserved communities. Indeed, South Los Angeles represents one of the most underserved communities in the country. Its residents need and deserve better health care. Working in partnership with others in the community, I believe I can make a meaningful and lasting contribution to improving the health of this community and reducing its health disparities.

I'm pleased to move back to the provider side of the health care system at a time when delivery system reform is one of our nation's most urgent imperatives. I look forward to building a hospital that will leverage health information technology and process innovation to make care efficient, high quality, patient centered and integrated with other providers who serve the same patient population.

In terms of personal growth, I'm thrilled to have the opportunity to leverage the management expertise I've gained and the relationships I've developed over the past 20 years to build and lead a health care organization. And finally, I'm eager to help widen the cracks in the glass ceiling that, even today, allow relatively few female physician executives to become CEOs of hospitals.

So, as I move into this new and challenging role, I recognize the sizable risks of this change, but I am optimistic that the rewards will outweigh the risks. If you check back with me in a few years, I'll let you know how it turned out.

CHAPTER TWENTY

Enduring Leadership

by Barbara Le Tourneau, MD, MBA

My early career was a progression from an emergency room clinician to physician executive via an MBA. As opportunities for more and varied leadership responsibilities presented themselves, I moved from part-time into full-time administrative roles—starting in private practice group management, then health plan administrative leadership, and back to delivery system executive positions. Within these organizations I was able to learn the healthcare system from the administrative perspective of physicians, health plan and hospital.

Participation in several national organizations including the American College of Physician Executives, The American College of Healthcare Executives and the National Association of Managed Care Physicians augmented my administrative work. I received a number of awards and certifications.

Mentors were key to my development as a manager. I had several important mentors, some male and some female who gave me advice and opened doors for further education and experience. My early management career advancement was covered in the 1995 *Women in Medicine and Management: A Mentoring Guide*. In this updated version, I will focus on my evolving view of leadership including future leadership opportunities.

SOUL SEARCHING 1

In the late 1990s while working as the Vice President of Medical Affairs

(VPMA) of a region of a Twin Cities integrated delivery system, I went through a divorce. Like so many women with full-time jobs I had depended on my husband for support at home. Suddenly I had two young children and no partner. Losing that relationship and unwinding a marriage forced me to rethink my life including my goals and priorities for the future.

Many of us face similar turning points—the loss of a spouse or partner, as mine was, the death of a parent, children leaving home or a personal health crisis. What I learned from my own experience is that stopping to take stock of one's life and career is important—even without a significant life crisis. As we age and mature, our life paths and views of life change. If we don't reassess with openness and flexibility, we may end up locked into unsatisfactory paths.

So when is the right time to take stock? In my experience, it takes at least five to ten years—first in clinical practice and then in management—to acquire a good sense of the joys and tribulations of each. It also takes that long to appreciate what is important in life and career. When this happened to me I had been in clinical practice for almost twenty years and in full-time management for six years.

In the late 1990s, during the time of my reassessment, I was working as Vice President of Medical Affairs of the North Region of an integrated delivery system in Minnesota. The system resulted from a merger between an HMO with over a million members and delivery systems with several large hospitals and a large multispecialty clinic. At the time of the merger I was the Interim Medical Director of the health plan. After the merger, I took the VPMA job on the delivery side, working primarily with the two large community hospitals in the northern suburbs of the Twin Cities.

An interesting opportunity presented itself in 1998. I hired a consultant named Hugh Greeley to help with education as I reorganized the medical staff leaders of my hospitals. He liked my approach and invited me to work with him with other medical staffs. So once a month I was on the road, helping other hospitals do what I had done at my own hospital. It was fun and interesting to see how different hospital medical staffs functioned and what kinds of reorganizations they developed. I learned a lot from these other organizations while bringing my own experiences to them.

Consulting was a new form of leadership for me. One of the roles I enjoyed most was that of change agent. As a consultant I could work with other medical staffs and help them design and implement change. This occurred at about the time I was completing my term as President of the American College of

Physician Executives. National work as consultant and president of the ACPE introduced me to a new kind of leadership role. Rather than being immersed in the politics and struggles of designing and implementing change in just my own organization, I could work as a change agent and advisor, or coach, to many different organizations.

As I thought about it, this incorporated some of the reasons I had always liked emergency medicine. It was episodic and short term. Like an ER doctor, a consultant does not need to be immersed in the day to day change issues to provide a fresh eye and new ideas when a crisis occurs or when a different approach is needed. This role helped me maintain my enthusiasm and expand my perspective. As I assessed my life and career in the late 1990s, new ways to provide leadership became clearer to me.

By 1999 I had been in full-time executive positions for nearly seven years. Before that I had been in a half-time executive position in my private practice emergency medicine group for five years. As I spent more and more time in a corporate structure I found myself tiring of corporate life. There were several issues that made working in a corporate setting frustrating for me.

First, I did not see many physicians move into the highest senior leadership ranks of corporations, and women physician executives were certainly not going there. Those physicians I did see in corporate senior leadership, while capable, tended to be part of the male bonding system. Nationally, I was not seeing corporate senior leadership ranks populated by individuals with diverse views, such as women and non-Caucasian men. There were many opportunities in hospitals and group practices, but few if any at the corporate senior leadership level.

Second, while physician executives were asked to engage physicians in their organizations, a majority of senior management did not take them seriously when they actually presented these physician needs. As a physician executive, hospital or corporate leaders often expected me to bring physicians into line with hospital or corporate goals. My suggestions as to how to accomplish this were often minimized or ignored. When someone on the management team made a misstep, ignoring my advice to avoid an activity or strategy, I was expected to manage and appease the unhappy physicians.

While I had many opportunities to implement what were very innovative ideas in 1999, the practice and frustrations of leaving physicians out of decision-making enhanced my dissatisfaction with physician executive work. I was never sure if the differences in philosophy were due to old-fashioned thinking on my part or too much business centeredness in high level management thinking. I suspect that many of my partners in management found it equally frustrating to work with me since I did not share their goals and principles in dealing with physicians.

In 1999 I decided to leave my full-time executive work and start a consulting company. I planned to work half time as a clinician in the ED and half time as a consultant, both in my own company as well as for Hugh Greeley at The Greeley Company. Because I was marrying again in 2000, I knew I could rely on my fiancé's full-time job for health insurance benefits for my children and me once my COBRA benefits expired.

Throughout my executive career I had always maintained some clinical practice. My specialty of emergency medicine allowed me to pick up a few ED shifts here and there. I realized that I still thought of myself as an ED doc and that I still enjoyed touching the lives of patients and their families. In the late 1990s I recertified my Emergency Medicine Boards and worked very occasionally in the ED. I still had clinical skills and drive to help patients more directly.

As a result of self examination I decided that it was time to make a leap from full-time executive practice into my own business as a consultant. Although I am not entrepreneurial by nature, I came to see myself as a bit of a risk-taker. I happily left my full-time job and regular paycheck with full benefits for two part-time careers as a consultant and a clinician.

A LITTLE VARIETY PLEASE

During this time of my life I found many leadership opportunities—both professionally and personally.

Consulting allowed me to be a change agent, coach and mentor. As I returned to part-time clinical practice, I suddenly realized that to take care of patients at times of crisis requires definite leadership skills. The ED physician advices and coaches patients and their families, helping them deal with many problems of acute and chronic illness. In addition, I continued some national work for ACPE and began serving on several non-profit boards of directors. These activities provided different leadership opportunities I had not yet experienced.

Outside of my professional life, I discovered personal ways to provide leadership through volunteer activities. I developed new skills including becoming a master gardener myself and then teaching others to be successful gardeners, composters and environmental stewards.

It wasn't until late 2000, as I wrote for national publications, spoke on national platforms and held national positions as a way to build my consulting practice that I finally realized I am neither a marketer nor an entrepreneur. At first a surprise, I began to acknowledge the obvious: I have never been good at selling things. I don't have the instinct for setting up and closing a deal. I certainly am not good at selling myself and I do not have the drive to build my own business. However, as is true for many physicians, I don't act like a 9 to 5 employee either. Because of this, more and more of my consulting work has been from my independent contractor relationship with the Greeley Company and not through building my own personal practice.

One downside of leaving a full-time management position was the loss of certain perks. For example, my organization had always paid for me to attend several meetings a year. Now I had to pay my own way. However, building a consulting practice requires high visibility at these national meetings. It is expensive to market oneself and requires a special kind of savvy or even pushiness. I learned that my strength was in leadership presence, not in drumming up business or marketing myself.

SETTLE INTO SOMETHING

At the end of 2001 a recruiter contacted me about a VPMA position for a local hospital. I knew that outside recruiting for a hospital VPMA job in the Twin Cities was rare, as most hospitals that are part of large systems tend to recruit internally. As it turned out, this was a hospital where I had often worked as a medical student. Suddenly, the idea of finishing my career in a familiar place was appealing even though I had not been considering taking another full-time executive position.

It had been two years since I had worked in a corporate setting, but I had been in many hospitals as a consultant. I was happy with my half-time consultant, half-time clinician work, but the paychecks were variable and I was interested in being home every night. So I interviewed for the position and felt that the hospital president shared my philosophy about the roles of physicians. I became the new VPMA in early 2002. As a bonus, clinical work in the ED was part of my contract. I was also able to maintain a small consulting practice as long as I used my own vacation time when I had to travel during business hours.

I was excited to be in a more concrete leadership role again, eager to bring lessons learned and ideas discovered in my consultant role, to lead a hospital and medical staff of my own. Although it took time to learn the medical staff systems and culture, I was eventually able to introduce a stronger medical staff leadership system, bring a new method of physician peer review and work with nursing and various specialties to design systems introducing evidence based practice into the hospital.

Having strong medical staff leadership has always been one of my core beliefs. Strong physician leaders are needed to come to the table with the management team to advocate for the needs of their patients as well as the needs of physician colleagues practicing in the hospital. If physicians can learn to speak with one voice, whether employed or independent, they are more likely to be heard. This became a primary goal for me as VPMA. It was also an important principle in my consulting practice.

I was very happy in this role, despite the inevitable corporate bureaucracy that delayed many of the programs I hoped to initiate. Once again, as a hospital executive, I was working not only within a hospital, but also with a large medical group and a health plan system, trying to manage their disparate interests. I particularly enjoyed the influence I could bring to system level projects.

In late 2003 the hospital president who hired me retired and within a few months a new hospital president came on board. Unfortunately he and I did not have the same vision of physician involvement that I had shared with his predecessor.

In 2004 I sensed the focus shifting to a stronger corporate identity with more emphasis on corporate needs and less on the needs and involvement of practicing physicians. It seemed that corporate quality initiatives were decided at an executive level, with assistance from executive physicians, but without the involvement of medical staff leaders. After the decision was made, the practicing physicians were expected to follow the program and I was expected to make them do so at the hospital level.

I learned more about my nature as a leader in this VPMA role. I realized that I am unable to lead in a direction I don't believe in—something I should have understood in 1999 when I left my last full-time management position. Now I saw more clearly that I couldn't set aside my personal beliefs for the good of the job. Perhaps if I had been more skilled at expressing those beliefs to the corporate leaders, I may have succeeded in shifting their thinking. However, I believe my personal values and ideals versus those of the corporate leaders were too different to reconcile.

In late 2004 I left the corporation and returned to consulting and clinical practice. I remained on the hospital staff and continued to practice in the ED. I still had my clinical skills and the desire to help people as a clinician. My departure from my VPMA position was amicable and there were no issues with my clinical ability. I had maintained a consulting practice with the Greeley Company and also with my own small company. Luckily, my husband's work covered my health insurance.

Within a few months of leaving any job, it is important to do some self-analysis to discover patterns and lessons. When I did that, in my own "ahah" moment I realized that I had left each full-time executive job after three to five years. That seemed to be how long it took for me to understand the particular organization and become successful as a leader there before I found the work to be too routine. At that point, I stopped growing as a manager and became frustrated and even negative about the job. Whenever my dissatisfactions outweighed the benefits, I became less effective and either had to leave the position or put aside my principles and needs.

SOUL SEARCHING 2

In 2005 my life, once again, took an unexpected turn. My husband, who was in the army reserve, was activated in the spring and deployed to Iraq. During his deployment I had my own two teenage children and my teenage stepson living with me. A younger stepson lived with his mother. The children living with me were old enough to pitch in and help with household activities, but not old enough to stay at home alone when I traveled or worked overnight.

Once again I had to prioritize. Since my income was larger than my husband's, I had to continue working. Luckily, we had the resources to hire help for cleaning, shopping, errands and driving. In addition, my mother stayed at my house when I traveled. I had to develop a new set of leadership skills, helping my husband's children cope with his absence while coping with it myself.

Things changed dramatically again in 2006 when my husband was killed. Once again a life trauma led me to seriously reassess what was important. Because the army took good care of the children and me after my husband's death, I was able to take three months off to adjust to the changes in my life.

I was nearing the final five to ten years of my career. How and when did I want to end my career, and how did I want to live the rest of my life? I began to realize that, for better or for worse, leadership and influence are engrained in me. I also recognized that I am unable to sacrifice my principles for the good of a job. Moreover, I now understood how important clinical practice was to me.

ENDURING LEADERSHIP

Because my husband died in the line of duty, the children receive military health insurance coverage through college. I am covered for the rest of my life. This freed me from having to take a full-time job for health insurance benefits. Although I could have retired at this point, I still wanted to work and felt I had something to offer both as a leader and change agent and clinician.

As I prepared to return to work in late 2006 an opportunity presented itself— a recurrent theme in my life. The Greeley Company needed more full-time consultants. They asked me to consider a leadership position in the company. I was not ready for that level of commitment or another full-time corporate position, but agreed to the role of senior consultant as a half-time employee. I was also able to continue my clinical practice, moonlighting at several hospitals.

In my consultant role, I work with many large and small hospitals as advisor, confidant, coach and change agent. I focus on helping medical staff develop into stronger leaders. Sometimes this is accomplished through education and sometimes by modeling leadership behavior. My best role is that of change agent, as it was when I had full-time executive positions.

I am not involved in the leadership of The Greeley Company. This works for me since I have learned that corporate politics and influence at that level is personally frustrating. It brings out a tendency for me to resist change rather than shape it. Also, as a consultant I do not have to work in a corporate office, giving me more freedom and control. I am much happier being an employee under these circumstances.

The same is true in my role as clinician. I now work at only one hospital. Working part-time helps me better tolerate my frustrations when dealing with both the healthcare system in general and the individual difficult patient. I plan to retire from clinical practice in May of 2012 when my last hospital medical staff appointment expires. I have been in practice for thirty-two years. Changes in clinical work are getting harder for me and I believe it is better to leave early with your skills and reputation intact.

As I consider full retirement I think a lot about enduring leadership and how one can keep it alive. I have done a lot of work on non-profit boards and find that type of leadership extremely satisfying. Volunteering as a physician is another possibility. Part-time consulting suits me as well and may meet my need to continue to provide leadership, helping medical staffs shape the changes they will have to adopt.

Bottom line: As has happened so often in my career, an opportunity seems to come along just when I need it. Who knows what will happen next?

PHARMACEUTICAL INDUSTRY

CHAPTER TWENTY-ONE

Doing Well by Doing Good

by Ellen Strahlman, MD, MHSc

Introduction

"Life can only be understood backwards, but it must be lived forwards."

— *Soren Kierkekaard*

When I was asked to be a contributor to this book, I was taken by surprise, as it is not my habit to look backwards. What inspires me in life is the possibility of what comes next, what problems to solve, what adventures to undertake, what joys to experience. I was even more surprised when, looking back in detail, to take an accounting of the good fortune I've had in my life and my career. It has given me a healthy dose of gratitude and perspective.

Although first trained as a public health physician, I've spent most of my working life in the pharmaceutical industry. Over the past 21 years, I've worked with thousands of extremely bright and talented people, most of them passionately dedicated to making life better for the millions of people their efforts touch. In industry, nothing is accomplished without teamwork, and the most successful teams have the twin goals of the pursuit of excellence and the ambition to serve patients. It has, and continues to be, a privilege to work with my colleagues, and to serve society as part of our industry.

But my good fortune at work pales in comparison to the good fortune of my life and the people closest to me. I've been married to two very accomplished men, both physicians with their own notable careers, and despite differences that led to eventual separations, they've been very present as fathers and step-fathers to our children. My children and step-children have all grown up to be talented, thoughtful, ambitious and caring people who are making their mark on the world, hopefully having gained 'something good' from their loving, complicated and restless female parent (me). During my training and throughout my career, I've been helped and mentored by many extraordinarily talented people, and benefited greatly from their wisdom and generosity. And my small intimate circle of family and friends are the source of strength, energy and light in my world.

So what follows is the story of my professional life, so far. It's not a perfect story, certainly not a story I planned in advance, and I have no idea how it will end. But I hope you find through the words and deeds, the ups and downs, and twists and turns, a life I sought to lead to help people, a life that leaves the world better than how I found it.

Early Life

I can't remember a time that I didn't want to become a doctor. One of my earliest memories is at age 5. Sitting on the table in my pediatrician's office, asking him how to use the reflex hammer that made my leg jump! The TALMUD says that "the highest form of wisdom is kindness" and if that is so, my childhood pediatrician was very wise. He was the soul of patience and gentleness, his eyes twinkling through his thick, slightly smudged glasses at the curly-haired inquisitive child who didn't stop talking during the entire examination. According to my father, so many questions were asked that day, he told my parents to send me to medical school to find the answers!

During my childhood, my mother suffered from the ravages of what we now know as manic-depressive illness: joyful, energetic, full of life on Monday.... quiet, withdrawn and absent on Tuesday. It is difficult to remember a breakfast with Mom. While she could not seem to get out of bed in the mornings, she was always there in the afternoons. The golden-haired beauty of her large, extended family, she would describe 'the sadness that never ends' to her eldest daughter, with a tragic poignancy that touches my heart to this day. Her suffering made me feel helpless, and I wanted to become smart enough, skillful enough, to help her. Knowing that doctors help people who are unwell, I wanted this to be the work of my life, to help people, with the knowledge, compassion and kindness shown to me by my pediatrician.

Growing up in the late 1960's and 70's was a time of substantial civil unrest in the United States. Tensions in my mixed-race schools in the Long Island suburbs often kept us out of the classroom. During these years, I learned lessons of tolerance and the terrible consequences of inequality: Black friends who walked with me in elementary school became distant, militant and sometimes violent adolescents, and many of them never finished high school. From these years, my values of fairness and equality emerged, laying the foundation for the belief that no person should be deprived of essential human rights, and that governments should take care of the basic needs of all their people, especially healthcare.

My questioning the world around me and my desire to understand how it worked ignited a love of science as a youngster. And the passion for helping people through medicine grew stronger during adolescence. However, my family was not wealthy, and my dream of becoming a doctor would not have been possible without scholarships for both college and medical school. Despite many criticisms of the American educational system, it is possible to earn the opportunity for a great education, through the foresight and generosity of others, and I had the good fortune to benefit from this chance.

As an undergrad at Harvard, biochemistry opened up the fascination of the emerging fields of molecular biology and genetics; and many classes in applied mathematics unlocked the reasoning power of my mind. The application of mathematics to any problem taught me how to represent issues, how to frame problems, establish boundary conditions, and develop iterative lines of attack.

I treasured my medical school years at Johns Hopkins, some of the best time in my life. I absolutely loved the study and practice of medicine. The School has a long tradition of patient-centered care and research, and as students, we interacted with patients from the very first year. We were also encouraged to apply our minds to research, in the laboratory or in the clinic. I met (and later married) my 'medical school sweetheart' during these years, and entered my formal training with optimism and excitement.

Patients, Public Health, and the Path to Industry

During medical school and surgical training, the new science of evidence-based medicine was emerging, as well as its application to medical care, medical practice, and the larger issues of public health. Several of my clinical research papers were published in medical journals during this period. As an ophthalmology resident, I had the opportunity to work at the Dana Center for Preventive Ophthalmology, founded by two world-renown physicians, the first program of its kind in ophthalmology. It was fascinating to realize the power of public health methodology to impact the lives of people. A colleague at the Center had discovered the link between vitamin A deficiency, blindness and diarrheal death, during his fieldwork. Here was the potential to improve the lives of people, millions at a time. This was a complete paradigm shift for me in the consideration of science, having done lab work or patient case series in my previous research.

At the same time, came an even more profound paradigm shift for me: the birth of my daughter in 1985. Once she arrived I knew, with sudden, certain and joyful clarity, that my priorities were forever changed. Of course she was the most beautiful baby, ever. I never wanted to have to choose between the urgent needs of a patient or my child. The joy of motherhood had taken its place in my heart—no job would ever be more important than raising my children. As I was pregnant now with my second child, I no longer desired a life as an academic surgical ophthalmologist . I was gratified to have support from my advisors at Johns Hopkins, men and women, who also prioritized family life alongside their careers. Between us we developed a strategy to pursue options for research fellowship positions in public health. Two of my professors from Johns Hopkins sponsored the application for an Andrew Carnegie Public Health Fellowship in 1987. Each year, two physicians with demonstrated aptitude and commitment to outcomes-based research and public health were selected for the fellowship which included sponsorship of a Masters Degree, a living stipend, a book allowance and a modest grant with which to conduct a research program.

The good news came in early 1987, and my mentors were thrilled: I was the first ophthalmologist, and the first surgeon, ever to receive this award. Knowing that the work would start in September of that year, almost on cue, a bouncing baby boy arrived precipitously into the world (6 weeks early!) in June of 1987. The fellowship consisted of obtaining a Masters Degree in Epidemiology & Statistics at the Johns Hopkins School of Public Health (1989), as well as clinical research, that was eventually published in the Archives of Internal Medicine in 1990. This work identified a gap in access of ophthalmic care among the indigent population in Baltimore, despite the presence of a premier eye institute at Hopkins. As a result, a vision screening program was installed in the General Access Medical Clinic, with the ability to immediately triage a patient to the Wilmer Eye Institute.

After the completion of my fellowship, I accepted a position as Senior Medical Officer at the National Eye Institute (NEI) in Bethesda, Maryland where responsibilities included the design and conduct of epidemiologic research and clinical trials for ophthalmic diseases, particularly age-related macular degeneration and myopia. In addition, I led a series of two-day workshops addressing access to healthcare issues (building on the work of my Masters'

Thesis), bringing together stakeholders from industry, academia, policy and the community—this was my first experience in expert consortium-building—a skill that would serve me well in the future.

It was an exciting time to be at the NIH. Almost everyone, in one way or another, was caught up in the furor of the AIDS epidemic, and the work to find the cause and cure for HIV was well underway. During my Masters Degree studies, I developed a keen interest and expertise in clinical trial design, and this allowed me to become part of a special Task Force comprised of colleagues from NIH, FDA and academia. We examined the possibility of applying clinical trial designs for drug testing that would allow medicines to reach patients faster than ever before. This work laid the foundation to what would become the 'expedited pathways' for drug development in the future.

It was not easy to balance the needs of a family and a career, and my marriage suffered, even as work and the children were flourishing. The change in family circumstances that eventually led to a divorce left me uncertain as to how to continue my career. The expected path was back to a university appointment, where I could see patients, do surgery and pursue research. Not an energizing prospect, given the long on-call hours that would be required for both clinical work and research. Conditions had changed for academic hospitals by the early 1990's, and many academic ophthalmologists spent most of their time generating revenue instead of pursuing high quality research. As I was contemplating what to do, a call came in from a headhunter—my first experience with recruitment—inquiring about my interest in a role in industry.

I had not even considered the possibility of working in industry, but went for the interview anyway. It was fascinating to think about drug discovery and development, and the analogy to public health was very compelling: a new medicine could save the lives of patients, millions at a time. The experience in HIV showed me the urgency of patients' needs. This was true in many areas of medicine; and I realized for the first time the potential contribution a pharmaceutical company could make.

What 'sealed the deal' was meeting the people at Merck, where I started my career in industry. These were some of the brightest, most passionate and dedicated people I'd ever met in medicine; many were from academia, and they were determined to find cures for the diseases they were researching. The role nearly doubled my government-based salary, would not require weekend and nights on-call; so it seemed a perfect solution for my mind, my heart and the balance of my life.

From Expert to Manager and Understanding Teamwork

Joining industry in the early 1990's was not a career path of choice for most physicians, and it was not easy to persuade my parents and my mentors in academia that this would be a good option. For my parents, it represented turning away from patients and a predictable life-style; for my colleagues in academia, it was giving up scientific principles and objectivity for business interests. They were wrong, not only about me, but about the hundreds of thousands of people who work in the pharmaceutical industry. And I was sure for myself that I need not, and would not, give up these ideals.

Joining Merck in 1991, my initial responsibilities were in the area of ophthalmology, my greatest area of medical expertise. This included support for development programs for glaucoma, particularly a novel carbonic anhydrase inhibitor program, dorzolamide (Trusopt). The Trusopt program was in a state of disarray, having completed no less than 22 Phase II studies to ascertain optimal dosing and formulation activities. The Phase III program was well underway, and at several centers, an allergic response to the medication had been observed. I was asked to lead a safety analysis of this apparent adverse response, and present my findings to Senior Management. Following this presentation which included a substantial grilling from the President of R&D, it was agreed that the program could continue. Best of all, after only nine months in industry, I was asked to lead the team that would complete its development!

As Program Director, I led a matrix team of 50, coordinating all departments in the completion of the regulatory dossier. This was my first real experience in management—in the past, relying on expert knowledge and ability to work with others was my contribution to the work. This was a very different set of skills: my colleagues were all experts in their area, and we had to organize ourselves to get the work done, with the deadline in mind. The responsibility of the program leader was to analyze different components of the work, then propose a plan to achieve the desired result. This required not only a new strategy for the program, but a re-alignment of the team to the new goals and objectives, which included negotiation with the FDA and European Regulatory Agencies. We were successful, and the study results were also positive for patients, The global dossier for dorzolamide was filed in February 1992.

With this accomplishment, I earned my first promotion, to Director. More important, however, was learning the value of teamwork in solving complex problems. This is not an easy psychological shift for many physicians—in medical school and in taking care of patients, physicians often see themselves as the keeper of expert knowledge, strongly guiding decisions, directing others. In the pharmaceutical industry, when leading a team of experts, different skills are required to ensure that everyone's skills and knowledge are applied to achieving a result.

Understanding the value of teamwork made future responsibilities easier to undertake. In addition to continuing responsibilities for Trusopt and CoSopt development, the scope of my position was expanded to include all medical marketing launch preparation activities for both products which included internal and external meetings with colleagues in all of Merck's major markets, worldwide. For the first time, I worked closely with colleagues from other countries and cultures, a tremendous learning experience. Trusopt was approved in the US in January 1993; in the EU in May, 1993; and the product was launched in that year. During this time, the CoSopt (combination of timolol and dorzolaminde) Phase II program was also begun.

After the launch, however, I became intellectually restless: having devoted two years exclusively to ophthalmology programs, wanting to apply my epidemiology skills and previous experience in HIV to work outside of ophthalmology. This is one of the great aspects of working in industry—the ability to work across therapeutic areas and disciplines—since discovering and developing a medicine requires so many different skills. Most of the work in industry is conducted by cross-disciplinary project teams, so it is possible to be exposed to, and contribute, on many levels. The success of Trusopt gained me a reputation for achieving results in a team-oriented, constructive and timely way, an organizational talent that was recognized by my supervisors and others within the company.

Expanding Horizons... in More Ways than One!

It had been a thrilling prospect to see a medicine come through the regulatory process and become available to patients. At Merck, we were advancing in our progress in developing medicines for HIV, very close to my heart after my experiences at NIH. It was an exciting time to be in the pharmaceutical industry.

In 1993, I married again, and we were now a blended family with 5 children between us, ranging in age from 5 to 21. My step-children had lost their mother several years earlier, and the transition was not easy for any of us. There was a lot of love in our home, this grew among all of us over time and continues to this day; and our international eclectic family uses all available means of communication and social media to stay in touch.

Also during this year, I was promoted to Senior Director, and joined the Epidemiology Department at Merck. This role was responsible for all outcomes research programs for products in the Ophthalmology, Neurology, Infectious Disease and Endocrinology therapeutic areas. In addition to being intellectually fascinating, this was ground-breaking work in those days, the first time 'outcomes research' was systematically applied to late-stage drug development programs. Now I was part of the team, not its leader—and I learned just as much, if not more, by this change in roles. The experience demonstrated to me that teams succeed when the leader sets the vision, creates the environment and resources to get the work done; and individuals take personal ownership for their part of the work. When all this occurs, we can serve the greater good; in our case, bringing a new medicine to patients. This was the birth of my grasp of 'servant leadership' which has been the philosophy for my leadership style ever since.

By early 1995, the outcomes-based models for the CoSopt program were completed; and the negotiations with FDA were successful and would lead to approval. In addition, our teams developed the pharmaco-economic models, ensuring a 'break-even' price for Crixivan (for HIV), which became the basis for the model used for Fosamax in its later development. We also supported the Global Outreach Group in its financial modeling for the free distribution of ivermectin for onchocerciasis ("River Blindness") in Africa. So I had the best of all worlds in this role: working in ophthalmology drug development, outcomes research for HIV and participating in a philanthropic global health program— 'doing well by doing good' was very much in evidence during these years at Merck.

From Manager to Leader, and 'Servant Leadership'

During this time, Bausch & Lomb (B&L) was searching for an ophthalmologist with pharma experience to be the company's Chief Medical Officer. As often happens in industry, headhunters call with interesting opportunities. I never wanted to leave any role that I had, but the chance to go to a role that captured my imagination and had even greater problems to solve on behalf of patients was a very compelling proposition. Our family circumstances also made such a move desirable, and the role seemed to be an opportunity to put all I'd learned into practice—as an expert, a manager, a leader, with responsibilities that spanned an entire business. So I accepted the job in February, 1995, and left Merck on good terms.

At B&L my responsibilities were those typically required of a Chief Medical Officer of a pharmaceutical and medical device company: media and investment relations activities, all ethical and safety queries, final sign-off and review for all development programs and first-in-human protocols. In those days, B&L

also had Dermatology, Hearing, Sunglasses and Animal Health businesses. As CMO, I had similar oversight responsibilities in these areas.

This was my first experience in a Corporate role, where I was expected to lead and make decisions across a variety of functions and businesses. None of these areas reported to me, from an organizational perspective, even though I had the accountability to take the decisions and ensure they'd be implemented. So I was able to put the principles of 'servant leadership' to good use: I spent a lot of time talking with colleagues, outlining a vision for what we needed to achieve, gaining alignment, then going back to Corporate for resources and funding. There was a lot of energy, interest and positive intent from my colleagues; my focus was to capture this and create an environment and support plans for our work together.

In addition to the CMO duties, I was asked to directly supervise clinical development programs in the contact lens and pharmaceutical divisions, and to chair the technical review and implementation committees for these groups. As B&L combined its research, development, regulatory, and process scale-up operations from its three contact lens businesses, I led the integration of these groups into the corporate site in Rochester, New York. During this restructuring, I was promoted to Corporate Vice President, Medical & Scientific Affairs—the youngest Corporate VP in the history of the company.

This new role retained the media, investor relations and supervisory responsibilities over all medical and development activities for the company. For the Pharma Division, this included three Phase III programs, and for Licensing and Business Development, we participated in the acquisition of two leading ophthalmology surgical companies: Storz Ophthalmics and Chiron Vision. After the deal closed, integration was needed for the research, development, and regulatory affairs for both companies into B&L's structure and sites. As this work drew to a close in early 1998, I was asked to move to Pharma Headquarters in Florida to lead the Global R&D Groups for this Division and became Corporate Vice President, and Global Head of R&D for the Pharmaceutical Division in Tampa.

While maintaining responsibilities as company CMO, the new role included direct oversight of all research, development, regulatory, process scale-up, and medical marketing activities for the B&L Pharmaceuticals Division. There were sites in Tampa, Florida, Pearl River New Jersey and Berlin, Germany. At the time, B&L Pharma in Tampa was the premier liquid generics manufacturing operation in the US, producing more than 200 products for the US market in the areas of ophthalmics, otics, inhalants, nasal sprays and IV medicines.

The other half of the organization was Dr Mann Pharma in Berlin Germany, the leading provider of ophthalmics and nutraceuticals in Germany.

These were exciting years during which I learned about the development and distribution of generic medicines. The outstanding teams working on these products accomplished a great deal, including bringing to the market more than 30 generic medicines (ophthalmics, nasal sprays, otics, inhalants and IV medications). Approval of the proprietary programs, Azelastine, Lotemax and Alrex ophthalmic NDA's also occurred during this period. In Germany, 12 new nutraceutical programs were launched and the New Jersey Discovery Group completed two deals leveraging chemistry from large pharma companies for ophthalmic drug discovery. Finally, Phase II program for the drug delivery technology, Retisert (fluocinolone implant for uveitis) was initiated.

Although the Pharma Division was profitable for B&L, the company decided to re-structure and downsize the division in 2000 in order to re-focus its efforts on its core businesses (contact lenses, solutions, surgical). This heartbreaking re-organization included dismantling the Discovery Group, moving all ethical programs, including the Retisert platform technology, back to Rochester; and a reduction in the Tampa and Berlin workforce. During my six years at B&L, we'd re-structured at least eight times. Although it was interesting and exciting to combine and consolidate businesses, there is a considerable human toll, since all of these changes necessitated people losing their jobs. This was not easy for me to do—it still isn't—and I grew very weary of it during these years.

At the same time that the company was undergoing transition, my family was experiencing change. During my B&L years, I'd traveled often to the UK and other parts of Europe, and had begun considering a move there. We'd always wanted our children to study abroad, so as the company was re-structuring, it was agreed that I would support the transition of my responsibilities, with a plan to leave B&L by the end of 2001, the same year our two youngest children began their studies in UK schools. This was a bittersweet time, even as the children embarked on this new adventure because my husband and I separated. I left for the UK to a new role that promised to be exciting, but with personal uncertainty and very mixed feelings.

From Large Pharma to Biotech

In January 2002, I was invited to join Virogen Ltd as its Chief Executive Officer. After ten years of larger corporate life, the opportunity to lead a small energetic group of people with brilliant ideas seemed a refreshing change.

Virogen was a biotech company specializing in proprietary technology in the virology area, with compounds for Hepatitis C, Hepatitis B, RSVand HIV. In addition, the laboratory was uniquely equipped to conduct live viral assays required for target verification, and earned credible revenue from contracts with large pharmaceutical companies. The business model was a hybrid of revenue generation (from the lab) and medium-risk development (Phase II and III programs). As a business spin-off from the Medical Research Council for Technology in the UK, the company had received seed-capital from the MRC. Now, it was seeking funds to capitalize the business model to progress the programs and create an independent company. In my role as CEO, I had responsibility for all business operations including, business strategy, fund-raising and investor management, medical, scientific, commercial, manufacturing, contractual obligations. However, my most important activity was fund-raising—the quintessential lesson from my experience in biotech. It took three months of intensive VC (venture capital)-shopping throughout Europe (the usual 24 firms in 12 weeks) before we received two initial term sheet offers for capital—both at a substantial premium. After completing a financial analysis and evaluating alternatives, the Board voted to consider selling the assets of the company as a greater return on investment as well as a more secure route for employment for its employees. We ultimately sold the major assets of the company to Arrow Therapeutics, also based in London.

Having responsibility for a biotech company that specialized in viral illnesses that plagued developing countries also gave me exposure to many issues facing global health, and the potential contribution of the pharmaceutical industry to address these issues. This led to a consultancy assignment to CoreRatings, a firm specializing in Corporate Social Responsibility ratings for large and small companies. The result was a co-authored sentinel report entitled "Corporate Social Responsibility in the Pharmaceutical Industry", outlining the issues, remedial actions and value-added steps for biotech and pharmaceutical companies.

From R&D to Commercial

By the time the deal closed in May, 2003, I had received a job offer from Novartis which was planning to acquire the ex-US rights to Lucentis from Genentech. Having a taste for working with VC's and business development, combining my R&D and commercial skills in such a role was intriguing. So I agreed to go to Novartis as Senior VP, Head of Global Development for the Ophthalmology Business Unit based in Basel Switzerland. This was perfect timing for my family, as my children had two years to complete their education in the UK before starting college.

The Global Development Organizations within the Novartis Business Units were fully integrated Early/Late Development and Medical Marketing Organizations, with groups in Switzerland, Japan and New Jersey. Since Novartis Ophthalmology had licensed several products from partners, this was my first in-depth experience working with colleagues from other companies to develop and commercialize medicines. The cultural differences between countries and companies made communication a challenge at times—and working through these issues gave me a tremendous appreciation for the perspectives and needs of other types of businesses.

The teams developed and commercialized many important products for patients during these years, particularly therapies for 'wet' (neovascular) age-related macular degeneration, the most important cause of blindness among the elderly populations of the developed world.

However, the seemingly endless re-structuring that plagued B&L was now pervasive in our industry, and my time at Novartis was no exception. During the first four months, major re-structuring was needed for the R&D and Medical departments, simultaneously, at both the European and US sites. In early 2004, Novartis announced a merging of the Specialty Business Units (Ophthalmology, Oncology and Transplantation). Part of this re-structuring included a complete dismantling of the Ophthalmology Discovery group. I was disheartened by this, realizing this would significantly slow down our pipeline efforts for Ophthalmology.

Also during this time, my youngest children were completing their high school studies and were ready to start college. The divorce had taken its toll on our family; my daughter wanted to return to the US for college studies and it was important for me to be close to her during these years. Fortuitously, I was offered a position at Pfizer as the World Wide Therapeutic Area Head for Ophthalmology in 2005, and decided to return to the US to take up this role.

When I joined Pfizer in March, 2005, the company was contemplating a re-structuring of operations from a site-based organization into a Therapy Area (TA)–based organization. Mine was the first joint role in both the R&D and Commercial Organizations, charged with the responsibility of unifying the therapeutic area across the complex matrix and site organization within Pfizer. The responsibilities included directing research and development efforts for ophthalmology as well as global medical and commercial direction and lifecycle planning for all Pfizer ophthalmology products and portfolios worldwide. The business responsibilities included all early and late stage product development programs as well as global and US medical strategies, content and input. In addition, I was the therapeutic area lead for licensing and new business development for Ophthalmology. In a little over two years, Ophthalmology at Pfizer completed three external licensing deals and three drug delivery platform technology deals to supplement the pipeline. The company now had programs in Glaucoma, Dry Eye, AMD and diabetic retinopathy. The internal development pipeline program grew from one program to twelve during this period; many of which were from substrate within the Pfizer R&D portfolio.

As the Medical Head of the therapeutic area, the responsibilities included representing Pfizer Ophthalmology to the global medical, scientific, academic and regulatory communities as well as interfacing with World Health organizations (e.g.,International Trachoma Initiative). In addition, my departments were actively engaged in academic and industry collaborations for the advancement of medical knowledge for Ophthalmology in the areas of biomarkers, translational medicine, genomics, molecular profiling, and drug delivery. Overall, Ophthalmology at Pfizer now had a 'footprint' of more than 500 colleagues worldwide (excluding manufacturing), and we were now an established, productive and profitable part of the Pfizer portfolio and business.

While at Pfizer, I was also involved in a number of company-wide initiatives, as the company continued its transformation under the leadership of its new CEO. This work included interactions with colleagues in the Business Development organization at Pfizer. Happily, these efforts were appreciated, and the challenge of optimizing the portfolio assets within the R&D portfolio, as well as a consideration of upgrading our strategies for in-licensing activities, was invigorating. I was invited to join this organization in August, 2007, and I welcomed the opportunity to apply my R&D, medical and business knowledge to the company's plans for asset acquisition.

I joined Worldwide Business Development in August, 2007, with two sets of responsibilities as VP: Out-Licensing for all of Pfizer's Therapeutic Areas and In-Licensing for roughly half of them. Out-Licensing was a new function for Pfizer, a new department needed to be created, and it was expected that we would eventually partner or externalize both de-prioritized portfolio assets as well as tail commercialized products. My Search and Evaluation (S&E) colleagues led teams that completed deals or acquisitions with the following companies: CovX Pharmaceuticals, Coley Pharmaceutical Group, Serenex Inc, AVANT Immunotherapeutics, Benitec Ltd, Encysive Pharmaceuticals, and Chiesi Farmaceutici.

Turning 50:
a Time for Reflection

Toward the end of 2007, I turned 50, and this became a salient moment for me. Although I was not particularly sentimental about such milestones in the past, there seemed to be a 'convergence of change' in my life at this stage and it gave me pause.

My children were now in their college years and my step-children all employed and satisfied in their various life/work situations. They were my priority for time and emotional energy outside of work for many years, especially working through the changes in our family circumstances. Now that they were happily embarking into adulthood, their needs changed, all for the good, and this was a big change for me.

Now there was more personal time for friends and intimacy, and this expanded my sense of participating in the larger society. I realized that I'd focused mainly on work and children in prior years, and the shift into 'the world out there' re-activated my interest in many areas. I started playing the piano again. The kids and I learned how to scuba dive (not an obvious activity for a confirmed claustrophobic!) and we actually took more real vacations together.

A less positive change was caring for my parents, who had reached their late 70's, and were experiencing more health issues. In helping them, my interest in healthcare delivery and the larger issues of global health were re-ignited, and I began thinking about how I could participate more fully as part of my working life.

There was now a range and depth of experience that I could to apply in a larger context. Although it was a tremendous experience to have re-built a therapeutic area and work in Business Development, once we'd identified potential technologies, a lot of my time was spent analyzing financials and future sales. Becoming more involved with the health issues of my parents drew me back to issues of medical practice, contact with patients, and their context of care. In considering the many projects and programs over the years, some succeeded, but many more failed, for both predictable and unpredictable reasons.

Most importantly, I'd become keenly aware of the profound reputational and environmental challenges that our industry was facing, and would continue to face in the years to come. Despite the long history of accomplishments and contributions of the pharmaceutical industry to global health, the manner in which business was conducted was under intense scrutiny. The now-famous 'patent cliff' loomed large in the plans and risk management strategies for many large companies. There seemed to be the very real possibility that the potential of our industry's longevity was at stake—that its future contributions to society, from humanitarian, development and financial perspectives, would be at risk if things did not change. At the same time, despite tremendous progress, global disease and public health issues were increasing, so the need for new medicines, vaccines, healthcare infrastructure and delivery was also growing.

I wanted to be part of solving these problems, addressing issues inside the large companies and working with stakeholders outside the company to ensure the continued progress of global health for society and assure the success of our businesses in the future.

As the year 2008 unfolded, I was once again restless for change, craving an opportunity to bring a more expansive, holistic, patient-centered approach to my work, and hoping my diverse portfolio of experiences would allow me to serve in a role that would be meaningful and highly impactful for our industry and for the society.

From Leader to Servant:
Inspiring Change through Authenticity

In the spring of 2008, GlaxoSmithKline (GSK) approached me about joining the company to become their Chief Medical Officer. This was an incredible 'convergence'of life and work! The CMO at GSK has accountability for all matters of patient safety and medical governance for all of GSK's businesses (Pharmaceuticals, Biologicals/Vaccines, Consumer Health, ViiV), and serves as the senior 'medical voice' for the company in matters of external engagement. The company's leaders were looking for a physician, with experience in industry to oversee three broad areas of activities: medical risk management, organizational change, and an interest for matters of global health. There was a great 'meeting of the minds' during the interview process and I joined the company in the summer of 2008.

I was the first woman to be appointed to be the Chief Medical Officer for a large pharmaceutical company. But it is a testament to our time, and the success of many senior women leaders in the pharmaceutical industry, that this was not a major issue for me, nor the company, when I was appointed. I did not feel unusual or unwelcome in this setting –both Pfizer and GSK have notable, very accomplished and very talented women among their senior ranks. And, I might add, the same is true for my male colleagues

As the Chief Medical Officer for GSK, I had oversight for all global medical, regulatory, safety, compliance, quality, medical advocacy and access policy functions for the company. The work included the pharmaceutical, vaccines and consumer health businesses for the company. At GSK, the CMO is accountable to the Chairman of the Board for all matters of patient safety, general medical governance, ethics and integrity, medical information, and investigation involving human subjects relating to any GSK products in development or on the market. The CMO is also accountable to the Chairman of R&D for all pipeline governance safety matters. In this role, I served as management member of the Board Audit & Risk Committee; Chairman of the GSK Global Safety Board, Medical Governance Executive Committee and R&D Compliance Boards; Member of GSK Senior Management Committees including the Product/Portfolio Investment Board, Scientific Review Board, Technology Investment Board, R&D Executive Committee, and Vaccines Global Health Forum.

A particular pleasure for me was to be invited to join the Board of Directors of ViiV Healthcare, plc, when the company was formed in 2009. ViiV is a joint-venture company between GSK and Pfizer, designed and dedicated as a business to serve the present and future needs of HIV patients, all over the world.

Activities and accomplishments of the organizations under my watch included management and execution of responses to product safety and reputation issues across all business areas and key products including more than a dozen key brands, well known to the medical community. As Chair of the Global Safety Board (GSB), we reviewed the safety considerations for all major regulatory filings for the company, made recommendations and decisions for nearly every new program, and investigated many safety and risk management programs for products already on the market. The Safety Board also reviewed and approved many business development deals within GSK.

My teams were also responsible for strengthening, codifying and embedding the Medical Governance Framework across GSK. With senior leaders from all over the company, we gained the alignment and cooperation of all business units to this effort; leading and delivering the successful close-out of many regulatory inspections (including FDA, MHRA, others). We established the expanding role and remit of Medical Affairs within GSK and clarified the governance accountability for medical colleagues across all of our operating regions. In 2010, Global Quality and Compliance organizations was added to the scope of my responsibilities, and our teams extended the work of codifying governance activities to these areas.

Along with these responsibilities, my attendance on the Board Audit & Risk Committee, mad me appreciate the vast array of risk management activities that must be managed within a company the size of GSK.

Although I had always valued teamwork, communication, and collaboration in the past, my skills in these areas grew at a 'step-change' pace in this role. To inspire change in an organization of thousands of people required engagement in a very different way, both operationally and emotionally.

Operationally was fairly straighforward, requiring strategic planning. Many hours of talking and communicating with colleagues, in small settings and large ones. Regular video meetings with colleagues from all over the world. Visits to leadership teams and colleagues from across our diverse businesses and regions. And even a blog—to the great amazement of my children and their friends!

The emotional perspective required looking deeply inside myself, to connect to the purpose of what I was doing, in order to share it effectively. In many areas of our company, colleagues would need to embrace a new way of working in response to our external environment and to correct some errors of the past. New rules, new constraints, new policies and procedures are never easy to swallow. More importantly, a new mind-set was required to make this happen. What I realized for myself, is that if these things changed, we would be able to continue our great contributions in bringing new medicines, vaccines, products to people that would improve their health and well-being. I knew that the vast majority of my colleagues were also deeply attached to this mission and purpose—these ideas brought many of them into our industry—so I sought to capture this sentiment, this purpose, this intent, for myself and others—and connect it to the work that needed to be done. And it seemed to work. We've made tremendous progress, accomplished a great deal during these past 4 years, and the work continues.

From Inside to Outside:
Including the Whole World in Our Work

During the summer of 2011, decisions were taken to re-structure the role of CMO in light of a change in leadership for Pharma R&D, as well as other corporate matters. The new role was envisaged to have a much greater emphasis on product safety and pipeline delivery, and several of the organizational components were diverted elsewhere. During the first three and a half years with GSK, there was much to be done for medical risk management, product defense and organizational change. There had not been much time to invest in global health or consider our external stakeholders, other than handling product safety matters.

GSK has a long tradition of contribution to Global Health, and strategic discussions were underway to raise the scope and ambition of our work in these areas. As my role was being changed, given my background and passion for this area, my CEO asked me to create a new Corporate Capability for Global Health Initiatives with an emphasis on Neglected Tropical Diseases. For me, this would be the opportunity of a lifetime!

Taking on the leadership for GSK's activities in Global Health, particularly Neglected Tropical Diseases, is perhaps the deepest expression yet, of my personal journey to positively impact, as much as possible, the lives of patients, millions at a time. And it is an incredible opportunity to enhance the contribution of our company, to include the whole world in our work.

This new role continues to evolve, and includes oversight of GSK's humanitarian drug donation programs and community partnerships, Senior Executive Advisor to the CEO Future Strategy Group and PULSE Program. I also remain on the Board of Directors of ViiV Healthcare and continue to be the Executive Sponsor of the Vaccines Public Health Forum.

Particularly energizing in this new role, is the privilege to represent the company in many medical matters relating to public health, access to medicine programs, and other external engagement efforts. Some examples include working with recently-created United Nations' Commission on Life-Saving Commodities for Women & Children, participating in a healthcare workshop sponsored by the International Centre of Missing & Exploited Children, Healthcare Coalition and various NGO partnership programs.

So What Happens Next?

Throughout my life and career, I've aspired to live by the principle of 'doing well by doing good'. For me, there is a tremendous convergence in applying innovation, commerce and ambition to serve the greater good of society. I've been blessed to experience this in all aspects of my career: from becoming a physician, to studying epidemiology and public health, through supporting and leading the work to bringing medicines to patients, and most recently, working with many colleagues and organizations to improve the overall condition of global health.

So rather than writing a 'conclusion' to this account of my professional life so far, perhaps it is best to describe how it feels to be here, now. I will resist the temptation to give advice, hoping this reading provides some insight to the journey of a woman, a doctor, a mother, a pharmaceutical executive, and an advocate for global health.

An insatiable curiosity, the restless desire for solving problems, the joys of accomplishment, the opportunity to work with people who love science, medicine and who want to make the world a better place...this is the great privilege of my working life. Though I have never been one to take a prescribed path, the path I chose was the right one for me. It enabled me to maintain my focus on family while still feeling connected to medicine, to patients, and wanting to make a difference in their lives. Whether it is one at a time as an individual practitioner, or 'millions at a time' through public health and the pharmaceutical industry, it is tremendously rewarding and worthy work.

But this has not come without sacrifice and setbacks. Although the foregoing is mainly an account of the specifics of my career, there were, and continue to be, many challenges of working in my chosen profession and handling the life outside of work.

For work itself: I became a physician with a deep desire to help people, expecting this to be a rewarding and well-regarded profession. I was not prepared for the declining reputation of physicians, the healthcare system and the pharmaceutical industry that has occurred over the past twenty years. The business-driven consolidation of many companies which often requires downsizing of organizations, takes a profound human toll on the people working and the people who remain. I will never, ever, get used to having to tell people who are performing well that they have to leave a job for business reasons. And despite the great privilege to work at the global level, the physical impact of years of international travel is daunting.

The challenges are greatest in personal life. Time spent with loved ones may be cut short or changed at the last minute and the overall level of stress and exhaustion sometimes prevents the full enjoyment of moments we have together. The strain within a marriage or partnership, when both have active and ambitious careers, takes its toll on intimacy. Activities I greatly enjoyed in my youth—playing music, going to plays and concerts, dancing, sports— were difficult to maintain during the busiest periods. These challenges are shared by both men and women, and for me, I've come to realize that it's not necessary to 'have it all', but it is important to strive for the clarity, the joy, the fulfillment and the balance that works for you.

Life is a great journey and I think of myself as a 'realistic optimist' for both work and life. When I think about all that science, technology, communications, and globalization could offer every single person on the planet—with my head in the clouds and feet firmly on the ground—I truly believe the best is yet to come, for medicine, for our patients, and for our world. And if I continue to listen to both my head and my heart when making future life decisions, I am quite sure the best is yet to come for me as well.

ENTREPRENEURS AND CONSULTANTS

CHAPTER TWENTY-TWO

Cardiothoracic Surgeon to Entrepreneur

by Kathy E. Magliato, MD, MBA, FACS

I used to think that being one of the few female cardiothoracic surgeons in the world made me unique amongst my surgical peers. I now know that this is not entirely the case—even though the number of women who have achieved board certification in cardiothoracic surgery numbers approximately 200 since the inception of the American Board of Thoracic Surgery in 1948. In fact, it wasn't until 1961 that the first woman was able to attain board certification is this very male-dominated field.

It is, however, even more unique for me to be a practicing cardiothoracic surgeon with an MBA as I have yet to meet even one, other than myself. I am confident they exist, especially in light of the fact that undergraduate schools are now offering dual MD-MBA degrees. In fact, my own alma mater, Union College, in Schenectady, NY offers a Leadership in Medicine program in which students can obtain a BS, MD and MBA in an 8 year academic track. With hindsight being 20/20, I cannot imagine why a physician would not embark upon an academic path that ultimately leads to degree in business.

Having said this, my very own path to an MBA was a bit circuitous, and yet there was a certain convergence between getting an MD and getting an MBA. In the most simplistic terms, my motivation to become a doctor was so that I could heal people and my motivation to get a degree in business was so that I could heal more people. At the time I applied to the UCLA Anderson School of Management (the only school to which I applied), I was the Director of the Mechanical Assist Device Program at Cedars-Sinai Medical Center in Los

Angeles where I was enjoying my practice as a Heart Transplant Surgeon. I had, in fact, founded and built the Mechanical Assist Device Program using little more than my clinical skill set from my fellowship in Mechanical Assist Devices at the University of Pittsburgh Medical Center.

While building this clinical program and working with various artificial heart manufacturing companies, it became apparent to me that something was missing in my life as a heart surgeon and program director. In fact, that "something" was a language barrier that I simply couldn't cross—it was the language of business. While I was fluent in the language of medicine—a complex language grounded in science, theory and case study—I was completely ignorant of the language of business, a language also grounded in science, theory and case study. While one language was used to save lives, the other was used to change lives and I found them both extraordinary and necessary to my evolution as a physician and surgeon.

And that is how I found myself, at the age of 40, going back to school to take exams, write essays and spend 40-hours-plus per week "hitting the books". Unlike medical school which was rote memorization, business school was taught by the Socratic method and you'd best come to class prepared to lead a discussion of the latest economic debacle or Harvard Business case study or risk personal humiliation.

I found business school to be a great intellectual challenge. It was like a springboard for my mind. I found myself in a new territory of learning and exercising muscles in my brain that I never knew existed (and, anatomically speaking, do not exist). I also found myself surrounded by some of the greatest minds I have ever met—my fellow Executive MBA classmates. I learned as much from them as I did my highly proficient professors and it was all very stimulating, especially coming from a field of medicine that revolved more around a technical skill set.

All of this hard work and study certainly paid off. I finished my MBA in 2006 with a new cadre of assets, the two greatest of which were:

- The ability to build and leverage myself as a brand (and recognize the importance of doing this)

- The network of UCLA staff and alumni with whom I can collaborate and look to for advice and support in any endeavor I choose

---

Note: a mechanical assist device is an artificial/mechanical heart that can be implanted in the chest and replace the function of the human heart in a patient with severe heart failure. It can be used as a bridge to a heart transplant in a patient who would otherwise die while waiting for a donor heart to become available. It can also serve as a permanent implant to stabilize a heart failure patient.

Also, as a result of getting an MBA, I now address problems differently. I think differently. I act on my instincts differently. And most importantly, I am now constantly scanning my life for opportunity—especially opportunities that utilize both my business and clinical skills.

In terms of building myself as brand, upon graduating from UCLA Anderson I developed a marketing plan for myself as a physician and a platform that positioned me as a national expert in heart disease in women and women's health. To this end, I wrote a memoir, "Heart Matters", which was published by Random House and received a 4-out-of-4 star review from People Magazine. At its core, "Heart Matters" is a book that educates women about heart disease. Around that core of information, I added the stories of patients that I have taken care of throughout my career. The stories are both poignant and tragic and send the message to women that heart disease is our #1 killer and is an epidemic among women. "Heart Matters" is also a memoir of my life as a female heart surgeon who is juggling a career, two young children and a husband who is a liver transplant surgeon. In other words, a woman who is trying to find balance while trying to have it all and make a difference—isn't that what we are all trying to do?

I have leveraged this brand to build an extensive list of speaking engagements, radio, TV, newspaper, and magazine appearances and am currently working on both scripted and non-scripted projects related to my book and my brand. I would never have known how to navigate these marketing waters nor understood the power of brand-building and positioning had it not been for my business degree.

And yet, the most potentially rewarding project I am working on utilizes the second of the two greatest assets I received from my MBA—the ability to collaborate with and engage the Anderson community.

On the very first day of class, I met a fellow EMBA student with a PhD in bioengineering who was in the earliest stages of developing a cardiac diagnostic medical device. From that very first day onward, we collaborated on the development of that device with what little time we had outside of the classroom and MBA workload. We utilized the expertise of other classmates and professors to help us with things such as patent application, design development, and funding opportunities. Upon graduating from Anderson, we had built our business plan, patented the device and built a prototype. We have since completed the third and final phase of the prototype, performed safely and efficacy testing in humans and incorporated ourselves with the addition of a third member to our company. We have procured nearly half a million dollars in funding through US government grants and have given up no equity in the company.

Through this experience with my own med tech start-up company, I have become involved with 6 other medical technology companies in various stages of growth and am evaluating innovative funding opportunities such as the creation of a cross-border technology fund with China. All of which was made possible by networking with the UCLA community and beyond. I urge you, as prospective MBA students, to make the effort to really get to know your fellow classmates. Find out what they do for a living, what their passion is, and how they envision themselves in the future. You may be amazed by the synergy you have with them and by what a collaboration can yield. Also, stay connected with your business school. The alumni network will be an endless resource, teeming with opportunity and only too happy to work with you.

From my vantage point, I see an MBA creating a new breed of what I call the "entrepreneurial physician"—a physician who either creates new enterprises or uses their newly honed business skills to improve and build upon their existing medical practice. I fear, however, that doctors seek an MBA only to use it as a stepping stone to a position within health care/hospital administration and I think this could be potentially myopic. Once you get an MBA, change is in the wind, so keep your options open!

For me, the entrepreneurial route fit like a surgical glove. The high risk/reward ratio, the necessity of both speed and accuracy and the ability to exact more rapid change are the very "surgical" qualities of entrepreneurship that drew me to this field of business. And yet, I am still practicing as a cardiothoracic surgeon by day (and night!). I believe it is important for me to stay in the "trenches" of health care in order to keep my finger on the pulse of what is evolving in the field of medicine. In this way, I am able to convey real-time data to the companies I am assisting.

And so, for me, I will continue to use my MD to save lives one patient at a time, one day at a time and use my MBA to create technology that will change the lives of thousands. Either way, my hope is that I create a modicum of positive change in the world at large.

CHAPTER TWENTY-THREE

Creating Your Own Version of Success

by Kelly Z. Sennzholz, MD

Before I became a successful medical entrepreneur, before I was a medical manager and leader in various healthcare organizations, before I was an Emergency Room physician, I was a Registered Nurse. I still possess the tiny handprint of the first micro preemie I cared for, long before the word "micro preemie" was coined. The positive impact I was able to have on that baby's family is forever etched on my heart. I don't know if they remember, but I do. Working in the healthcare field as an RN, I was fascinated by the science of medicine. I found the ability to use science and complicated decision-making, in order to improve the lives of others, to be supremely interesting. As I moved into critical care and flight nursing, when those fields were quite new, it was truly breathtaking to be a part of the development of medicine as we now know it.

I worked in a hospital alongside some of the top nurses in the country including the author of a major nursing textbook who was one of the few nurses with PhDs at the time. Working with her, I realized that as you progressed in nursing you moved away from the clinical bedside and closer to research and writing. As I compared the jobs of the physicians I worked with to the PhD nurses, it seemed evident that being a physician was a better way to remain at the bedside. I took the chance and applied to medical school, receiving admission letters from two on my very first try. It was a new path for me, but one that held great excitement and opportunity.

The same day I began medical school, my son was starting kindergarten. I clearly remember standing there, he with his red and yellow briefcase schoolbag with large A, B, C's on it and me with my heavy backpack. wishing each "Good Luck" on our new path. We were both ready for a new adventure. I was a single mother, with a very supportive ex-husband and later, "wife-in-law", who made my life much easier. Still, it was quickly apparent that being a single working mother and going to medical school was something of an aberration in Oklahoma, even in the late 1980's.

I accomplished medical school in two parts: I finished the first two years of didactic material commuting to Oklahoma City, while I completed the two years of clinical immersion in Tulsa where I lived. The needs of my growing son were my first priority and affected every decision I made regarding my career. While I juggled mothering duties, work to sustain my son and me along with my medical studies, it never occurred to me that those without obligations like mine found simply being a medical student so onerous. Although at the time it actually seemed exciting and fun, I couldn't even tell you now how I did it all. The story of the oil that lasted for eight days comes to mind!

After medical school, I chose a residency in Tulsa in order to stay near my ex-husband. The medical school was just starting a Med-Peds program and since I loved pediatrics and had received the "Outstanding Student in Pediatrics" award, this seemed perfect. However, one year into the program the pediatrics department unexpectedly increased their on-call requirements. As a single mother, I felt I couldn't handle the increased call responsibilities and ultimately decided to leave the pediatrics portion of my training behind. An outstanding Emergency Medicine group in our city invited me to begin moonlighting with them. It was exciting and interesting. Moreover, it provided additional experience that helped advance my career.

At the end of my residency, I joined that group as an attending and clinical instructor. By the time I was 30, I had worked in a range of medical areas: pediatrics, neonatology, internal medicine and emergency medicine. Because of the changes in residency programs today with earlier specialization, few physicians have the opportunity to work in as many areas as I did—a change I believe is not good for medicine. For me, the ability to experience a real breadth of medicine has made for quite an unusual career.

Despite the outstanding on-the-job training I received from some of the best ER docs, I had come "of age" too late to be grandfathered into Emergency Medicine boards which limited my working in some of the larger academic institutions. So I moved to North Carolina where I found opportunities in Trauma Centers and ERs at smaller hospitals.

I was eventually offered the Director position for Emergency Services of a small county hospital. During those years I joined a number of professional organizations in which I held several leadership roles. I became a representative for the medical society, president of a medical society, board member for state emergency physician group, medical examiner, Regional EMS director during seven hurricanes, state child fatality task force member and more. For five years I was responsible for creating funding for a clinic for the working poor. I also created legislative successes in the medical genre in two states.

As I look back on these experiences, I realize that in my family of origin, we were taught that every citizen has a responsibility not only to forward their life, but also to give back generously. I considered these activities my way of "giving back", not necessarily a career enhancing move. Nevertheless, they did help my career—if not directly—then in subtle ways. I made lots of great friends and interacted with some exceptionally bright and talented people. From administrative positions, to medical society leadership, from grant acquisitions, to community activities, I was able to see medicine from all sides in these settings.

Ultimately several things happened to cause me to move away from the clinical aspects of medicine to a more business approach to my career. The first occurred as a result of my work with the state medical society. I thoroughly enjoyed the camaraderie of fellow physicians. However, as the years passed, I realized the society was doing little to combat what I felt to be the negative influences of medicine, namely the loss of an independent physician/patient relationship.

The second was the recognition that the care we (physicians) were providing was not necessarily optimal. I had begun learning about wellness medicine which suddenly made me view medical care in an entirely new light. One example which illustrates this was a patient who came in each month for a "pain shot" for osteoarthritis. Normally, I just gave him the injection and discharged him. But this day, I asked him what his doctor was doing to cure the problem Exercise? Weight loss and nutritional guidance? Supplementation? Physical therapy? He looked bewildered and said, "Vioxx." Unfortunately, symptomatic treatment is often the rule rather than the exception. For so many patients we are not addressing their core problems.

The third was the recognition that emergency medicine is a young woman (or man's) game. Looking down the road, I didn't want to be like the gray haired doctor I knew who was still working night shifts at age 65, taking abuse from drunk and belligerent patients.

As a result of these insights, I re-examined my personal and professional goals, trying to understand what had made me choose medicine initially and what parts of my career brought me real happiness. For many physicians, it is the exactness of science, the need to be "perfect" which drew them to the field. But for me, the most rewarding aspects of medicine involved making a difference and bringing joy and health to patients. On those days when I was actually able to change the outcome of someone's life, I went home full of energy and enthusiasm.

Once I had completed this self-assessment, I was able to determine the direction I wanted to go next. I decided to leave clinical practice and study business—not formally through a degree program, but "on the job"—much as I had in the Emergency Room.

Determined to start my own business and focusing on improving the lives of physicians and patients, I started a small aesthetics facility. Although the learning curve was steep and not always easy, ultimately I developed a successful wellness program, then expanded it to a program to teach physicians about wellness. This success led me to start a technology company, eMedical Mall, an ancillary services management system that physicians could use in their offices to save them time and increase their reimbursements. The experience of starting and managing my own company not only broadened my understanding of the business side of medicine and non-medical endeavors, but allowed me to work with experienced, high level entrepreneurs who taught me the in's and out's of stocks, options, management, fundraising and many other core skills of the entrepreneur. My new venture, OSL Medical also provides in-house clinic programs. It allows the office manager to significantly improve clinic revenues, patient satisfaction and overall results without disrupting normal clinic flow.

In order to hone my leadership skills as I developed these companies, I took lots of classes. I also read numerous books on business, entrepreneurialism and finance. I studied hard as I was learning. I asked a million questions of my co-developers. I was a sponge. I love to learn and because this was a whole new arena for me, I was primed to learn the old fashioned way: through trial and error.

One thing that made my progress much easier were the many mentors I found along my path. Receiving and giving support, friendship, advice and feedback are a major necessity for those venturing out into this interesting but challenging world.

My first real mentor was a powerful woman who was named one of the top 50 women of the millennium, was awarded the Presidential Medal of Freedom and honored upon her death by the president for creating a brighter future for all Americans. Wilma Mankiller taught me many of the first lessons I needed to have the confidence to try anything. Yes, I got lucky on my first mentor. However, wherever you live, there are literally thousands of talented, successful, generous and educated leaders who are more than willing to give of their time and talent to assist you in your transition. The only thing they will expect in return is that you take the relationship as seriously as they do. As my career has moved forward, I have been privileged to become the mentor for others coming after me.

I personally do not think that physicians who want to be entrepreneurs need to go back to school to get an MBA. Having the degree may be more helpful if you are interested in entering the corporate world. It will definitely help you understanding the concepts and verbiage of the business world. But it is not necessary for most ventures you may choose to start on your own. Instead, consider taking classes for bioentrepreneurialism which are not degree programs. These can teach all the skills needed to get started in a shorter time frame. In my area, the University of Colorado offers an excellent series on bioentrepreneurialism. There may be similar offerings in other areas of the country.

Another good way to develop as an entrepreneur is to start attending networking events for business people. In almost every city, high-level entrepreneurs have groups that meet to share ideas and receive input. These offer terrific opportunities to begin learning the behaviors and talents required for a successful business. Listen, listen, listen. Take notes. Ask questions. We have a group in Colorado called SOPE (Society of Physician Entrepreneurs) which also has an interactive online presence on LinkedIn. Find a group in your city, jump in and start swimming.

Probably the best advice I can give to any physician starting down the entrepreneurial path is to choose a small project first, set aside time to work on it, and just begin. When you reach challenges, identify quality people who can assist you. I am constantly amazed at how generous all the more experienced business people have been on my journey. I, likewise, give back in any way I can.

As I have traveled down my career path, my personal and social life has varied a lot. Sometimes, working a regular job and starting a business required my full attention. Other times, I have found streams of income which allowed me more freedom in my personal choices. It is okay to forego personal activities for a time while starting a business, but it is also helpful to get feedback from friends and family if this time away from socialization has become too long or too hard. Each individual is different, but creating an ongoing balance is important. That is the holy grail in entrepreneurialism. There is this mysterious "perfect amount" of family/private time which I doubt anyone ever achieves for more than a week! But getting regular exercise, carving out time for relaxation and spending time with those you love are key to making life worthwhile. Make sure you put these things on your calendar every week. Schedule them in just as you would schedule in an appointment with someone else. Remember, you are a someone, too.

In general, growing a career in 2012 is much easier for women than it was decades ago. Certainly younger men are much more accustomed to dealing with women in the workplace. When I began my career, people commonly questioned whether women should work outside of the home. Such a query would bring an incredulous look from most young women today. Not only do a majority of women now work, but they are starting businesses at a record rate. As more than half of the classes of many upper level educational systems such as law and medicine are female, women need to take on the challenge of learning leadership. Some leadership skills will not always come naturally for the feminine energy. Enhancing natural abilities of communication, empathy and dedication with the skills of guidance, leadership and power are going to be critical not only for the women and participants involved, but for our country and our world.

For the younger women still on their educational path, I would recommend stopping every month or so and formally reviewing what you have learned, where you are going and what areas you can improve upon. By making personal development a regular part of your life, you will avoid some of the plateaus and disappointments that can arise when living life on autopilot. By making this a habit, you will be developing the habits of champions, thereby improving your odds of having a championship life and a championship career. Find someone whose career represents where you want to go and ask them for mentorship and advice. Finding two or three mentors is even better. By having guidance and putting your time towards the growth and development of your own life you can achieve anything. By creating a positive framework for your business career, you will then be free to express your innate intelligence and caring. Part of what made my success in business was the same thing that made my medical career successful. Although I had little understanding or experience when I went into medicine, my intention was to do it and I simply figured it out as I went along. Likewise, in my business career, I envisioned my dream of what my life would look like and what my career would look like. I just jumped in and started swimming. I utilized my mentors, my learning skills and my excitement and the end result was success. Part of my desire to share this story is to provide some of the insights into the tools available to assist you with creating a new career. Keep your innocence and excitement, ɔut use the abundant resources of people and knowledge that are available to make it easier and to avoid time and money-consuming pitfalls.

My own future holds many new adventures. With financial success achieved, my dream is to really give back and improve the world in creative ways. I have been a co-founder of a political action committee, a co-founder of an international art colony, a founder of multiple charitable endeavors, board member of elite charities and other interesting side projects. I hope to expand upon my previous experience and be able to use my time and talents to focus on some urgent community issues. My life, as a physician, a mother, an entrepreneur, a political activist and a philanthropist has had a common vision. I think that Ellen Degeneres recently said it very well, "I stand for honesty, equality, kindness, compassion, treating people the way you'd want to be treated and helping those in need. To me, those are traditional values. That's what I stand for. I also believe in dance." Well said, Ms. Degeneres.

I warmly wish each of you the best of luck in your travels within and outside the medical world. Life is a journey to be enjoyed and you are still the best and brightest women on the planet. The world needs your input. The world needs your excellence. Don't be afraid to make a mistake; that is all a part of the journey. Laugh a lot, live fully and create your own version of success, not someone else's.

CHAPTER TWENTY-FOUR

A Road Less Traveled

by Deborah Shlian, MD, MBA

"Two roads diverged in a wood, and I-

I took the one less traveled by,

And that has made all the difference."

— *Robert Frost: The Road Not Taken*

I was fortunate enough to hear Robert Frost himself speak those words when my mother took me to a literary seminar at Johns Hopkins University. Although it was long ago (I was in grade school), I remember very clearly the message I took from that brilliant poet: it was okay to be different, to explore possibilities and options others might not, to "do your own thing". Growing up in the late 1950's and early 1960's, a time when family and career roles were still fairly rigidly differentiated by gender, this view required adjustments from parents, friends, and particularly school counselors who regarded nursing or teaching as much more acceptable careers for women than medicine. Indeed, the idea of career itself was "something to fall back on", to be dusted off should a husband die or family economics really get tight. Full-time wife and mother was the generally accepted proper role for a woman of that era.

Needless to say, I took Frost's words to heart, starting with aiming for a medical career early in life and then by taking various forks in the path as opportunities presented themselves. And that, for me, has made all the difference.

The first fork came at the end of medical school when I had to make a decision about specialty. In 1972, although there had been some brief mention of Family Practice as a new specialty, there were very few residencies in the country and even less guidance as to where to find them—particularly on the East Coast. So, despite my fascination with the concept of a "new, complete physician", I chose the road of least resistance and matched with a Hopkins radiology training program. It was a chance vacation to Los Angeles during my internship year that changed the course of my clinical career. My husband (we married in my junior year and his senior year of med school) arranged for a meeting with the head of Family Medicine at Kaiser Permanente. Our preventive medicine curriculum in medical school had included a comprehensive study of what was considered by many traditionalists to be a renegade operation (or worse, socialized medicine) i.e., a group model, Health Maintenance Organization (HMO). The notion of salaried doctors working in a prepaid multi-specialty group that functioned as a partnership was different if not heretical in the 1970's when the vast majority of doctors were in solo private practice. But my husband and I had found the concept more than intellectually interesting. It seemed to make a lot of sense and we were anxious to see the system up close.

Dr. Irv Rasgon was my first real role model and mentor. Chief of Family Medicine at the Sunset facility, he charmed us from the moment we met him. Irv was the quintessential Marcus Welby—he even looked the part. A great clinician, outstanding teacher and natural leader, he was passionate about Family Practice and Kaiser. "Why specialize and become so narrowly focused when you can be a Family Practitioner and take care of the whole patient?" he asked us. Irv took us on hospital rounds and his patients, from the very young to the very old, obviously adored him. Moreover, it was clear that his peers in other specialties respected him. When he offered us the opportunity to come to Los Angeles, finish our training as FPs and become Kaiser staff physicians, we readily accepted. I left radiology; my husband left ophthalmology; together we headed out to Southern California where we completed our training, took and passed Family Practice boards and joined the Southern California Permanente Group as partners.

Looking back, the ten years I spent as a clinician in the Kaiser group provided the kind of education in medicine and management that no didactic program in either medical or business school could ever provide. We were at the forefront of what has been nothing short of a revolution in healthcare—working in a fully integrated system that allowed us to deliver quality care (as much of the full spectrum of pediatric and adult medicine that was feasible in an urban hospital/clinic setting) without the stress of wondering whether our patients could pay for the care they required (what we know today as "managed care"). We had the advantage of being hospital-based, making our in-patients easily accessible during the day while we saw our scheduled outpatients in our offices which were located in the same building. Similarly, we could often grab "sidewalk" consults from specialists who worked down the hall or just upstairs—thus avoiding long appointment delays for our patients. Lab, X-ray and other ancillary services were a floor below—another efficiency. We were given a half day a week of "paid education time" which my husband and I used to teach residents at UCLA.

Medical students from both UCLA and USC spent one month electives at our Kaiser offices and I was even able to satisfy my clinical research interests with such projects as a study of "Screening and Immunization of Rubella Susceptible Women" published in JAMA. My department held regular quality assurance and peer review sessions; we developed clinical guidelines long before it was fashionable. From a quality standpoint, I believed then and still believe today, that the group model is an ideal way to practice medicine. Unfortunately, it is also extremely capital-intensive and in the kind of highly competitive market that characterized California even in the 1980's, some of the original idealism began giving way to market pressures. As a primary care clinician, I became increasingly frustrated at my inability to influence policy. I felt that front line physicians had the best perspective for identifying and correcting problems within the system. Yet despite the fact that legally the group was a partnership, in reality it was governed no differently than most corporate entities i.e. top down and the top physician leaders were almost exclusively specialists. For example, the chief of my hospital was a surgeon who often stated that patients did not care about having their own physician, that they were primarily motivated by easy access to the system and that any clinician—doctor, NP, PA, would do just fine. It didn't matter. Needless to say, this undercut the fundamental principles of Family Medicine—taking care of the whole patient and being able to provide continuity of care by the same physician. In fact, this chief refused to accept the validity of our early studies (later, a group out of Vermont published the same findings) showing that patients with their own primary care doctor had fewer emergent visits and less inappropriate hospital admissions—both a significant cost savings and quality improvement. Again with hindsight, I now realize that his intransigence on this and other healthcare policy related issues created an opportunity for me to take my next fork in the road; my husband and I both decided to leave Kaiser.

With no one to provide career guidance, we began investigating how we could use our skills and understanding of healthcare to have a greater impact on the system. I wrote several articles as well as a consumer health guide for a national health maintenance organization and we both spoke at various venues around the country about problems involved with the delivery of care in the managed care environment. During the first few months of my "retirement", we were persuaded to start part-time law school at Whittier School of Law in Los Angeles with the intention of developing an expertise in health policy and health law. However, not long after starting my first semester, I was recruited to a management position at the UCLA Student Health Service (SHS).

I became Director of the Primary Care unit of SHS which serves all 33,000 undergraduate and graduate students on the university campus. As many as

400 patients per day were being seen in our clinic—most of whom used Student Health as their only source of medical care. What attracted me to the position was the opportunity to take many of the lessons learned from the Kaiser system and adapt them to this setting. In particular, I wanted to change the orientation of Primary Care from essentially a triage area to a comprehensive ambulatory care facility staffed by clinicians competent enough to have admitting privileges at UCLA Medical Center. That meant letting non-board certified physicians go and hiring only well-credentialed Family Practitioners, Pediatricians and Internists—a process fraught with legal/risk management/ personnel issues that I had to quickly research and understand. In addition, I wanted to integrate our service with the outstanding teaching programs in the medical school. That required developing a new level of diplomatic skill, delicately balancing the egos and agendas of various departments within the school. But happily, within a relatively short time we had created an impressive educational and research program that helped to attract medical students and graduate students as well as superior clinical staff. Our quality of care, patient and personnel satisfaction all measurably improved.

As my administrative duties expanded, two significant issues surfaced which ultimately led to yet another fork in my career path. First, was the question of whether I could be a successful manager and maintain a clinical practice without compromising both. Increasingly, I felt caught between what I perceived as two equally important and demanding responsibilities. In the past there seemed to be consensus that despite the difficulties, one could not be an effective and credible leader of clinicians without concurrently having an active clinical practice. In fact, with the exception of a very few full-time regional medical directors, that is still the model Kaiser uses today for most of its physician administrators. On the other hand, in many other healthcare organizations, the role of physician executive has expanded so that those who wish to assume broad management responsibilities within these companies realize they must relinquish the clinical role, instead bringing the strong patient care background as a resource to a new, more comprehensive job description. Still, I must admit, for me it was not an easy decision, though looking back, it was one that has made all the difference in my success as a manager. As an executive who was also a physician, I was in the unique position of developing and enhancing collaboration and integration of the medical and administrative staffs in the daily management and operations of the organization.

The other issue had to do specifically with my expanding operational responsibilities. Up to that point, everything I had accomplished as a manager was achieved without the benefit of a formal educational foundation. For example, I was asked to develop a budget, but had never taken a finance or accounting course. I was asked to make staffing projections, but had never learned the kind of operations research tools needed to create a truly robust model. Without a working knowledge of the language and concepts of business, one becomes totally reliant on non-medical administrative personnel whose orientation to the bottom line may at least sometimes run counter to quality. This revelation convinced me to switch from law school to business school and in 1988 I completed an executive MBA program at UCLA's Anderson School of Management (with my husband, by the way).

Two things occurred as a result of the MBA program. First, my job description expanded to include policy formulation, strategic planning, broader budgeting responsibilities, contracting for outside specialty care, risk management, and helping to develop and implement a computerized patient record to capture data for outcomes measurement. I became part of the senior management team, attending meetings heretofore open only to the non-physician administrators.

Second, I began receiving telephone calls and letters from recruiters alerting me to other opportunities in medical management. Suddenly, I was advised that my experiences as both a clinician and manager in two managed care settings, coupled with my MBA degree, made me a strong potential candidate for many organizations looking to import that kind of expertise. Both flattered and curious, I decided to explore a few of these possibilities.

I had never worked with recruiters before and so had no idea what to expect. Someone would call my office, identify themselves as representing a particular job opportunity, then inquire as to whether I wanted to be considered as a candidate and if not, did I know someone else who might. Surprisingly, the recruiter often had minimal information about the organization, asked few relevant questions about my management experience and none about my interests and career goals. Moreover, when I did interview I often found the opportunity quite different from that described to me—from the nature of the job to the organization itself. It seemed clear that these recruiters were not serving their clients optimally; sending inappropriate or disinterested candidates is a waste of time and money. However, as I've come to learn, even negative situations can become potential opportunities.

As a result of these disappointing searches, I suddenly realized that an unfilled niche existed: full-service, comprehensive search consulting in the managed care market. True, there were plenty of people out there calling themselves recruiters. But no other firm dealing in that specific market had someone with my credentials. As a respected physician manager continually interfacing with the national medical community, I felt I could bring a unique perspective to searches. My credibility could further enhance a client company's reputation as I discussed available opportunities with prospective professional candidates. The other value-added component would be my willingness to develop long-term relationships with fellow physicians, guiding them through the search process—even putting some on the management career path initially, then mentoring them along the way. As I had personally experienced, no one in the search industry seemed interested in investing the kind of time (and thus capital) it takes to develop an individual executive's career, nor does anyone (as far as I know) have the kind of hands-on understanding of the talent pool to give appropriate advice.

Despite the sense that I could do it better, it took many months of soul searching before I actually took the next fork in the road, eventually making the career transition from physician manager to medical management search consultant. My position at UCLA was vested, I had spent almost a decade developing staff and programs I believed in including collaborations with both UCLA's Anderson School of Management and the School of Public Health, I loved working with the students and I had been told by my professors in the management school that more new businesses fail than succeed—especially consulting firms. According to an article in Fortune magazine at the time, only one new consultancy in five actually thrived. If I really wanted to be an entrepreneur, I had to be willing to take that risk.

Armed with a business plan including mission statement, I finally decided to take the plunge. Starting in 1993, I began to slowly build a firm that initially concentrated only on physician executive searches. As a career counselor to potential candidates, I often spent untold hours evaluating career goals, life priorities, reworking resumes, developing better interview techniques, and assisting with contract negotiations. The best payback has been the satisfaction of having launched many successful management careers, watching these individuals make significant contributions to a variety of healthcare organizations. Over time my clients began to request broader services, so I expanded my focus, becoming a consultant for various enterprises including established as well as start-up health plans, academic institutions, utilization review companies, research organizations, even other healthcare consulting firms. I have helped these organizations build high performance management teams by identifying appropriate entry, middle and senior level non-physician as well as physician management personnel vital for their success. That means fully understanding the organization, from governance to culture, evaluating specific personnel needs, conducting local and national salary surveys as the market changes, keeping close tabs on the interview process from start to finish including contract negotiations and following-up regularly with both the client company and new employee for at least a year after a placement is made to be sure an optimal transition has been achieved.

In 1994, my husband Joel joined me as President of the company. In 1998 we incorporated as Shlian and Associates, Inc., moving our main base of operations to Florida where we could help care for our aging parents. Both Joel and I stayed active in professional health care organizations such as the American College of Physician Executives and the Group Health Association of America, always keeping abreast of changes in medicine and in particular, managed care. We also regularly contributed articles and chapters for various textbooks on current management issues. Additionally, we developed affiliations with over a dozen associates with offices across the country, all with strong health-care backgrounds, who we could call upon to assist with specific searches. In this way, we were able to service our clients effectively while still maintaining the boutique nature of the company. Many small business owners feel compelled to expand in order to demonstrate success. However, according to Douglas Handler, an economist at Dun & Bradstreet, longevity rather than growth is the real measure of achievement. "Companies that last three years will usually make it," he claims. "Indeed, if you begin a company to capitalize on the wisdom and personal service of a key individual—namely *you*—big is bad. Adding staff and projects can spread the core value of your firm so thinly that customers are dissatisfied." David Birch, founder of Cognetics, an economic analysis company noted for its studies of small firms has said: "In the knowledge-based service firm, there are no economies of scale."

After over fifteen successful years, this worked well for us. We continued to enjoy repeat business from clients who hired S&A knowing we were much more involved in the details, we personally knew prospective candidates, and we could do the job more efficiently and less expensively than larger firms with high-rise offices and huge overhead. While a large firm might be able to coast on its reputation, Joel and I never could. If we performed poorly for clients, our business would fail. Bottom line: being your own boss is definitely not for the faint of heart, but if your vision triumphs, the success is yours alone and therefore all the sweeter. For me, the shift from a management position in a highly bureaucratic and hierarchical organization to CEO of my own company has been the most exciting and positive experience of my professional life.

In 2008, with responsibilities for parents' care accelerating, we made a conscious effort to slow down our consulting and recruiting business, traveling less and taking on fewer clients. At the same time, we renewed our interest in creative writing. Joel and I had collaborated on two successfully published medical mysteries while still living in Los Angeles (one with Simon & Schuster and one with Berkeley Books), but much to our agent's chagrin, never wanted to give up medicine or medical management to write fiction full time. Now we decided to finish a novel about China that we had been plotting off and on for years. That became "Rabbit in the Moon" and was published by Oceanview Publishing, a small hardback publishing firm that focuses on mysteries and thrillers. "Rabbit in the Moon" has won a number of literary awards including the Gold Medal for the Florida Book Award (we got to meet the governor); First Place, Royal Palm Literary Award (Florida Writers Association); and the Silver Medal for Best Mystery, ForeWord Magazine. The Audiobook version even won an Honorable Mention at the Hollywood Book Festival. Encouraged by this success, I have written two new medical mystery thrillers—"Dead Air" and "Devil Wind". Both of these were co-written with a former UCLA colleague, Dr. Linda Reid and have also won a number of literary awards. Joel in the meantime has developed a new interest in photography, which he finds equally creative, but with more immediate gratification (a novel takes years to write, then about eighteen months from the time it is sold until the publisher releases the print version; a photograph can be seen and appreciated right away). The most important lesson these endeavors have taught us is that physicians should develop interests outside of medicine so that the transition to retirement is not a loss of identity. Sadly, a number of our colleagues have sunk into depression the moment they are no longer called "Dr."

Finally, today, as I continue to mentor young physicians, I am always asked about the value of an MBA, particularly by those contemplating switching from clinical medicine to management. I can say with great confidence that for me, the MBA education and the degree itself have made all the difference in my career. As a manager, I was able to directly apply the classroom knowledge to my work, enabling me to expand my role to include much more of the business/ operations side of the organization. As a search consultant, I regularly work directly with CEOs, CFOs and COOs who appreciate the fact that I can speak their language. Often intimidated by physicians, they feel comfortable talking to a "fellow MBA". As the CEO of my own business, the training in accounting, finance, and marketing has been particularly useful.

Notwithstanding the value of a management education for me, I would advise any physician considering going back to school that an MBA will not provide the same kind of ticket that the MD did. By that I mean, having a business degree on your resume, even from one of the elite schools, is not sufficient to land you a job as a manager, nor is it still generally required for most positions. What really counts is management experience and the ability to show that you have produced tangible results for an organization, often identified by such measures as greater market-share, larger profits, decreased costs, reduced utilization, better outcomes and increased patient satisfaction.

An MBA should never be viewed as the means to "get out of medical practice". In fact, I would submit that if you really hate clinical medicine, medical management is not for you; it can be every bit as demanding and frustrating as clinical practice. Moreover, as the rate of change sweeping America's health care delivery system has accelerated, healthcare companies are reinventing themselves, developing competitive strategies that mean greater risk and more uncertainty than ever. Medical managers entering this brave new world, particularly those at the middle level, need to understand the landscape and be prepared to deal with it. Rather than one by default, the decision to be a manager should be a positive career choice. As the traditional separation of administrative and clinical matters is becoming obsolete, the modern physician manager must be a manager first and a clinician second. Bringing a clinical background to the new role of manager can certainly enrich the job, but does not substitute for specific management skills and training. Whether medical management as such will ever become a real recognized specialty is less important than the fact that only those who understand both the language of business and of medicine will be able to straddle the various camps that now control the practice of medicine in this country.

For me, the career path from clinician to medical manager to CEO of a management search firm has been anything but a straight one. With each opportunity came a choice and a certain risk. But in the end, it has been those forks in the road that have made all the difference.

CHAPTER TWENTY-FIVE

Six Lessons I Wish I Had Learned Earlier

by Kathleen Goonan, MD

I decided to go to medical school after spending two years exploring public interest law and government work in public health. My father was a first generation college student in his Kansas family who went on to become a pediatrician and physician executive. He was my first role model and I often tell people that if he'd been a restaurateur, I would probably have become one too. While I resisted following in his footsteps at first, I finally relented, even though it required returning to college level work to shore up my science background for medical school.

In truth, I've always been a leader and manager of systems. By nature, this is my talent: systems thinking and problem solving. I worked for the California Department of Health Civil Rights Unit before going to medical school. While in school I served as president of the American Medical Student Association. I chose primary care internal medicine for my residency because I wanted to have long term relationships with my patients and their families. The systems thinking aptitude drove me to opt for working with people and serving as the liaison between them and the health care system.

Little did I know when I made that choice how virtually incompatible being a full-time primary care clinician is with taking on the role of full-time physician executive—my ultimate goal. By the time I was almost through my residency, others realized this as well. Four months into my fellowship in health services research, I was offered a position as the medical director for a health plan affiliated with Massachusetts General Hospital where I had completed my residency.

Since that first position twenty years ago I have served as a senior executive at every stage of the health care 'food chain' from insurance to patient care delivery. Along the way, I've been fortunate to have not only my dad as a role model and mentor, but many of his physician executive friends as well.

My story is unusual. No one I know has become a full time administrator literally four months out of residency. Most move from clinical medicine to management in a slower progression. No matter how quickly one transitions into a leadership role, there are basic lessons common to all. I have decided to write this chapter as if it were a graduation speech as I look back on my life and career, sharing a few pearls I've collected (in addition to using generous amounts ofsunscreen at a much earlier age!).

Define your own, personal "true north" early and often

When I reflect on how and why I was able to develop leadership skills, I realize that it was only when I pushed the *pause* button, or after someone else encouraged me to push it and clarify *who* I was trying to become, that I moved forward and grew as a leader. I am not talking about job title or function, but about the values I believe in and which now, looking back, I am proud to have lived in my work.

For example, I have always believed in being a truth teller, even when that choice could cost me in the short run. As a senior resident, I was on a team that clearly erred and those errors in diagnosis led to harm to a patient. My fellow senior resident failed to appear at the Morbidity and Mortality Rounds. But I did and owned up to the mistake in front of the group. It hurt. I was scared. People didn't talk to me afterward, at least not right away, and not comfortably. I knew it was the right thing to do.

Refining true north periodically is about more than your personal values and behavior. It's about the type of work and roles you are best suited for. I was fascinated with measurement and analysis early in my career. I worked in the Quality of Care Measurement Department at Harvard Community Health Plan under Dr. Donald Berwick in one of my first positions. I partnered with Dr. Brent James in developing and delivering curriculum in this area. It seemed clear to me that this area of expertise would be critical to any leader of a health care organization. Today, this and many areas of administration and executive skill are much more sophisticated.

So, hit the pause button, evaluate your chosen path, and assess the skill development options available carefully as you supplement your medical education in these other areas.

Define your scope and deliverables

While I realize this is consultant speak (that's what I do full time these days), everyone does need to do this to be effective. Ideally, your organization and your boss give you a job description and assignments to help you define your goals and deliverables. Unfortunately, in my experience, this is often not the case.

The most effective executives are those who can clearly articulate the scope of their responsibilities and define what they will deliver in terms of results with milestones and timelines. In a sense, they are writing their future resumes with what they have accomplished before they accomplish it. Then of course, they deliver. As physician executives, we are considered "overhead" i.e. every moment we are not seeing patients costs the organization our salaries. Therefore, we must provide measurable value for our time.

Learn process literacy

When I had the great fortune to serve as a judge for the Malcolm Baldrige National Quality Award (2000-2003), one of my fellow judges from another industry (as they all were) called health care "the bastion of process illiteracy in the U.S. economy." What he meant by this was that we are still a cottage industry of individual professionals and we have yet to view all work, including leadership and management, in terms of processes. If you can't define your multi-disciplinary, cross functional work in processes, how can you hardwire, measure, and standardize work? How can you make it highly reliable and efficient?

I coined the term "process literacy" to refer to this major and critical shift in how we think about our work in health care. Leaders in the coming decades will think and work this way. It takes the ego out of our organizations, because it makes work less dependent on individuals and more likely to be consistently successful. Perhaps that feature is part of the resistance to making this change? Regardless, high performance organizations and leaders operate this way.

Build your self-awareness

We all have strengths and weaknesses as well as talents and personal demons. Every one of us. Highly successful leaders foster their personal awareness of these issues over time. This is a characteristic of highly emotionally intelligent people. This takes discipline and can be learned. In many companies, high ranking executives are provided personal coaches to help them accomplish this. You can create these relationships from people around you, or choose to hire your own personal coach.

See one, do one, teach one...

Remember this old rubric of medical education? Thankfully, it no longer applies in most clinical training settings. However, it still operates in administration. Leadership is learned by observing successful leaders and imitating them as opposed to didactic sessions sitting in a classroom or simulation lab. It also is learned through teaching others. I encourage you to evaluate your teaching options if you are interested in administration. As a supervisor, you will be expected to be a mentor to those who report to you. Take this role seriously and learn from your organizational development and human resources how to be an effective mentor. The skills required are typically not taught to doctors because we are thought to be "beyond" this skill. It's not true. Just because physicians have deep content knowledge doesn't mean we also know how to manage and mentor people. Those who become good mentors usually do very well in their organizations. They bring tremendous value that generally gets rewarded. People are more grateful for meaningful mentoring than they are for praise; although generosity in admiring genuine strengths of others is always a good attribute among leaders.

Learn to manage conflict

This is particularly hard for women. We tend to take things much too personally and get too emotionally involved in relationships with others in the work environment. Strong male leaders are often the best role models for learning to manage conflict. The sooner you learn to manage conflict by remaining detached and focusing on the situation as opposed to personal dynamics, the better off you and your organization will be. Successful leaders and managers are able to defuse and depersonalize conflict, allowing themselves and others to resolve conflicts with minimal emotional drama. If the priority is the patient, conflicts are a distraction and a waste. Leaders who keep the focus on the patient and effective work on their behalf, always rise above the fray in our stressful work environments. And more often than not, if someone is doing something that irritates or angers you, it's not personal. They are not doing it for you; it's who they are and likely they behave that way with everyone else as well. Develop a capacity to let conflict run off your back quickly and you will be rewarded by reduced stress and great respect from your colleagues.

For those of you who aspire to leadership roles in healthcare, the above few pearls will help optimize both personal gratification and contributions to your organization. Good luck!

CHAPTER TWENTY-SIX

Coaching – What's in It for You?

by Margaret Cary, MD, MBA, MPH

After reading about the many accomplished women profiled here, some of you may feel that you could use help with your own careers in order to move into leadership roles within health care. Working with a professional coach is one way to facilitate the process.

The term "coach" was first used at Oxford in 1830 to describe the tutors who "carried" their students through exams. The first reference to sports coaching was in 1831. Executive coaching has only been around for decades. As executives ascend the corporate ladder, colleagues providing constructive criticism tend to drop off. At the same time, those ascending the corporate ladder often become less inclined to listen to others' observations about their management and leadership skills.

Who do these executives have to give them honest appraisals, to help them consider options, to ask the questions no one else asks? That's what coaches do.

"A masterful coach is a vision builder and value shaper who enters into the learning system of a person, business or social institution with the intent of improving it so as to impact people's ability to perform."[1]

"Coaching is not telling people what to do; it's giving them a chance to examine what they are doing in light of their intentions."[2]

The International Coach Federation (ICG) defines coaching as partnering with clients in a thought-provoking and creative process that inspires them to maximize their personal and professional potential.

Imagine someone who is your curbside "consultant" for management and leadership challenges and learning. Someone who gives you his or her full attention when you speak, who asks you questions designed to help you figure out your own solutions. Someone who gives you honest appraisals, questions your motives and pushes back when constructive. Someone who is always in your corner, who shares articles, books, exercises and asks, "In what other ways could you approach that?"

That's what coaches do.

Through much of my professional life people have come to me for advice. I listened, occasionally asked for clarification, and then offered my solutions— emphasis on "my." Problem solved, on to the next. As a physician, I was trained in differential diagnosis. Patients came in; I listened to symptoms, considered signs, performed a physical examination and listed all diagnostic possibilities that came to mind. I used deficit thinking to eliminate them one by one until I arrived at a few options. I ordered additional tests to eliminate some of these and investigated the handful that remained until I arrived at the diagnosis.

Leadership and management don't work like that.

A friend recommended I work with her executive coach.

"Coach? What are you talking about? I'm not in competitive sports."

"An executive coach, an honest broker, someone who offers a different perspective and who can help you sort options."

"I don't think I need that. I have all the degrees I need and make my own decisions. I'm straightforward. I don't want to lose that."

She smiled.

So began my journey, from coaching client to coach (see chapter 3 for my personal story). As a coach today I work with physician clients by helping them look at alternative perspectives, considering positives and negatives of actions, so that they can make considered choices.

Non-physician career managers and leaders enter management in their twenties or early thirties. Their mistakes can be excused with "She's young. She'll learn. She has a good mentor."

Physicians generally enter management roles in their forties or fifties. Our management skills are compared with non-physician managers of the same age, but physicians haven't had two decades to make management mistakes. We've been too busy learning medicine and seeing patients. We make the same mistakes non-physicians make early in their careers. We're developmentally delayed. What we've been taught in medical school and residency is 180 degrees from many of the skills needed to be an effective manager.

For example, as practicing physicians we tend to be risk averse. Making a mistake as a clinician could cause someone to get sicker or even die. Our role as healers depends upon our being The Expert. On the other hand, taking risks is inherent in management and leadership.

Likewise, listening to alternate views is a critical leadership skill. Unfortunately, many physicians become so vested in their careers, in diagnosing illness and being healers that they find it difficult to listen to alternate views. As I was, many of my physician clients are proud of the fact that they are straightforward, pull no punches, and ask directly for what they want. Managers and leaders need to be collaborative communicators.

Some of those strengths we have as solo clinicians can keep us from developing other skills we need as managers and leaders. As an executive and leadership coach for physicians, I hold a mirror in front of them and ask questions to guide them in developing their own solutions.

My clients often ask for specific skills, how to manage their time, how to work with their bosses, how to manage conflict. As physicians, the most common challenge we have is learning to control our limbic systems, in order to avoid our automatic, unthinking responses.

Remember, you can lead from anywhere in an organization. You don't have to be at the top of the organization chart. You can also lead from below by working with your boss as a team. Authority is about titles and organization chart positions. Leadership is about integrity and being comfortable in your skin. You choose the perspective through which you view the world.

One of the issues that may discourage physicians from considering coaching is time and access. Coaching can be done in person, through Skype and over the telephone. With our erratic schedules as physicians we often find it easier to use Skype and the telephone, supplemented by in-person sessions every three to six months.

Unlike medicine, coaching as a profession isn't as regulated – yet. Last year the International Coach Federation began requiring coach-specific training in order to become credentialed. We're still in the early days of standardization and establishing requirements for coaches, sort of pre-Flexner Report status. So, what should you look for when you select a coach?

1. *Coach-specific training from a respected, reputable organization or from an organization that has been accredited by a reputable organization, such as the International Coach Federation (ICF).*

   When I decided to learn to be a coach I wanted a program associated with a top-tier university. At the time, Georgetown was the only program that showed up in my searching. I also wanted an in-person program, with interaction, rather than an online program.

   Coaching is not therapy, mentoring or consulting. If you think of therapy as archaeology, mentoring as advice and connections, consulting as others' solutions, then coaching is architecture. To follow that analogy, like an architect, a good coach works with you to help you construct your personal future, guiding you in reflecting on how you approach challenges. Just as when choosing a physician, you need to find the right fit. It's your engagement and it's your future. It is tempting to ask for advice and solutions. You won't own your decisions if you don't figure them out for yourself.

2. *Your credentialed coach should have had mentored, supervised coaching by a credentialed coach, as well as at least 100 hours of coaching experience.*

   Atul Gawande wrote about the importance of engaging a coach in his own career.[3] His coach was a retired surgeon with more experience than Gawande, someone able to observe his surgical skills and offer suggestions for improvement. In learning to be physicians, we start by learning how to interview patients. In the beginning it's overwhelming to probe for answers to sensitive questions, to insert ourselves into our patients' lives, even as we realize it's a privilege. Our learning curves are steep. Like learning to ride a bicycle, eventually talking with patients becomes second nature. As a consumer, would you choose a physician who hadn't been shown the correct way to perform a Caesarean-section or a gall bladder removal by an experienced surgeon and was observed by such experts until she/he got it right? In general, the more particular procedures we do as physicians, the better we get.

3. *Your coach should use techniques with evidence for their effectiveness.*

   Yes, evidence-based methods apply here. A good coach will keep current with management and coaching literature and will modify what s/he does, just as with medical practice.

Finally, how will you know if the coaching has "worked" for you? The best way is to get feedback from others, before your coaching session and after. The process takes months, much as learning any new skill.

Bottom line, Management 101 is hard. Leadership 101 is harder. Coaching continues to move me toward more authenticity, as client and as coach. The coaching approach works as a manager, a leader and a parent. We physicians are lifelong, eager learners. Those of us who wish to become managers and leaders can learn the necessary knowledge base and skill set, just as we learned anatomy and genetics, how to interview patients and take blood pressures.

Sometimes we just need a little help, someone we trust who asks the right questions to help us find our way. That's what coaches do.

You can view a five-minute video of Dr. Cary's presentation on executive coaching at the 2012 annual meeting of the American College of Physician Executives at http://youtu.be/653anCaWwNk and read her essays at www.thedoctorweighsin.com. Contact her at medleadership@gmail.com.

REFERENCES

1. Robert Hargrove, Masterful Coaching (Pfeiffer, 2002) 17.

2. James Flaherty, Coaching: Evoking Excellence in Others (Oxford, UK: Butterworth-Heinemann, 2010) xx.

3. www.newyorker.com/reporting/2011/10/03/111003fa_fact_gawande, accessed June 12, 2012.

FINAL WORDS

by Deborah M. Shlian, MD, MBA

The questions so often asked by women physicians aspiring to management is, "How can I enter the field" and "How can I move up the ladder?" The fact that doors to leadership in organized medicine have swung open is only half the battle. Women have to be willing to walk through those doors. The women profiled here are a diverse group. Some are nearer to the beginning of their management careers, others are midway and a few are close to or have already retired. Some are married, some are not, some have children, and some have none. Some are surgeons by training, others are primary care doctors. While each of the women physicians presented in the preceding pages is unique, working as physician managers in virtually every type of healthcare organization in the US, their stories share some common themes. I've put together several helpful tips from their experiences.

Be a Clinician first

With one exception, each of the women profiled in these pages began their careers as practicing clinicians and although most have given up their day to day management of individual patients as they transitioned into more senior leadership positions, it was their work as a physician first which gave them the unique perspective required to be an excellent healthcare executive.

Know Yourself

Before considering a transition from clinical medicine to management, do a thorough self-assessment. Clarify who you are and who you want to become as a person and as a leader. Examine your values and goals. Determine your strengths and weaknesses as well as what brings you the most satisfaction.

Effective leaders are lifelong learners

President John F. Kennedy once said, "Leadership and Learning are indispensable to each other," suggesting that an effective leader should always be open to new information and perspectives. This is particularly true for the healthcare system, which is constantly changing.

Look for ways to polish your skills, and use those skills as building blocks to move ahead. The physician manager today must have an understanding of the details of the business of health care, including finance, accounting, strategic planning, information systems, organizational behavior, human resources, and relevant legal issues. Although there is an increasing trend toward formal education, one way or another, if you aspire to management, you will need these skills.

And even if you have a formal degree, you will need to integrate your reading and study with experience. So take every opportunity to obtain practical experience within the organization. The medical world is full of committees, task forces, etc. that can offer exposure to administration, working with people and systems and problem solving. The Related Reading Section that follows contains recommendations by the contributors to this book.

Know your organization

To borrow a medical analogy, organizations, like organisms, are organic and have specific structures and functions. The structure of a medical organization would cover such issues as the type of legal entity, the mode of governance, financing, etc. On the other hand, the overall way a specific organization functions is affected by what is often called its "cultural climate." For example, how do professional and nonprofessional staff interact; what is the extent of bureaucracy and hierarchy; how much operational responsibility is given to physician managers? Understanding both these aspects of your organization is critical to moving ahead.

Network

Get to know people both inside and outside your organization who you can tap for information and support. Young people involved in team activities tend to develop this critical skill earlier than those focused on more individual, competitive endeavors. If you are not already a member, consider joining the American College of Physician Executives. ACPE's stated mission is to help ensure that physicians continually grow as individuals and become successful health care leaders. Today the organization has about 10,300 members. Less than 20 percent are women. Hopefully as more women seek leadership roles, they will see the College as a great resource for attaining their goals.

Take the initiative

Don't expect handouts. In the corporate world, upper management promotes people who find and seize opportunities. Actively seek projects to take on. If you see something that needs changing, develop a plan and present it to senior management. Whenever possible, take on projects that give you visibility within the organization.

Be a risk taker

Be willing to grab opportunities where and when you find them. Whenever you read profiles of people who have had high-level management positions in and out of medicine, you find that they generally got where they are by taking on new assignments. For women, having supportive spouses and families is critical. Creativity helps, too. For example, if you want to participate on a committee and accommodate family needs, suggest doing some of the work through conference calls (including video) and e-mail.

Reassess goals as you go

Goals developed when you first begin your medical career will likely need adjustment as your personal life circumstances as well as the business/healthcare environment changes. Some people suggest reassessing goals at least every 5 years. The time increment is less important than having the discipline to do it.

Learn to negotiate

If you're not convinced of the importance of honing negotiating skills, consider that you negotiate every day, whether you're resolving conflicts between you and your spouse or children, working out vacation schedules with other physicians or staff, or discussing treatment plans with patients and their families. In terms of moving up the management ladder, men historically have been better at asking for things they need in order to be more productive to get ahead.

Refining your negotiating skills and learning to achieve win-win solutions will maximize your leverage as a manager.

Select the right subordinates

If you're in middle management, the personnel you select will determine how well suited you are for a senior position, because senior managers are generally judged not by how well they do, but rather by how well their staffs do. Senior managers must have a clear vision of the future of their organization. They need to be leaders for change.

Find a mentor and/or role model

This is not always easy, but it can make all the difference in becoming a successful manager. Find someone you'd like to emulate and ask directly for his or her help. More often than not, that individual will be delighted to share their wisdom. As you move up in management roles, become a mentor yourself.

Summing up

Most people today agree that the healthcare delivery system in the US requires fundamental change. I am among those who believe that physician executives articulate in the language of health care policy and business are in a unique position to lead the needed reforms. I also believe that women should be among those leaders. Women now make up half or more of medical school classes and have moved into clinical areas traditionally off limits to women. The challenge for the future is for women physicians to also move into top management roles. I hope some of you will be among those women.

List of Participants

1. Florence P. Haseltine, MD, PhD
   Chief Everything Officer (CEO), Haseltine Systems, Inc. &
   Emerita, Director of the Center for Population Research.
   2181 Jamieson Ave 1606,
   Alexandria, VA 22314
   Florence@haseltine.com
   240-476-7837

2. Margaret (Maggi) Cary, MD, MBA, MPH
   Executive Coaching and Leadership Development for Physicians
   Keynote Speaking, Retreat Facilitation and Group Coaching (202) 403-1966 Email: MedLeadership@gmail.com
   LinkedIn | Twitter
   Credentialed by the International Coach Federation
   Springsteen's Leadership Actions
   Leveraging with Questions: The Leader's Edge Co-author, *Telemedicine and Telehealth: Principles, Policies, Performance and Pitfalls*

3. Ora H. Pescovitz, M.D.
   Executive Vice President for Medical Affairs, University of Michigan
   CEO, University of Michigan Health System
   Professor of Pediatrics and Communicable Diseases, University of Michigan Medical School
   www.medicinethatspeaks.org

4. Donna L. Parker, M.D.
   Associate Dean for Student Affairs
   University of Maryland School of Medicine
   410-706-7476
   dparker@som.umaryland.edu

5. Kathleen Yaremchuk, MD, MSA
   Chair, Department of Otolaryngology
   Head and Neck Surgery
   Sleep Medicine
   Henry Ford Health System
   2799 West Grand Boulevard
   Detroit, Michigan 48202
   Phone: (313) 916-3275
   Fax: (313) 916-7263

6. Eneida Roldan, MD, MBA, MPH
   former President and CEO Jackson Health System
   Assistant Dean for Student Affairs (Recruitment and Professional
   Development)
   Associate Professor, Department of Humanities, Health, and Society
   Co-Academic Director for Professional Development
   Herbert Wertheim College of Medicine
   Contact: eoroldan@fiu.edu
   305-519-1652

7. Patricia A. Gabow, M.D.
   Chief Executive Officer
   Denver Health
   777 Bannock Street
   Denver, Colorado 80204-4507
   Patricia.Gabow@dhha.org

8. Jayne McCormick, MD, MBA
   Chief Medical Officer/Central Delivery System
   Presbyterian Healthcare Services
   505-841-1689
   jmccormic3@phs.org

9. Hoda A. Asmar, MD, MBA, FACPE, FACHE, FACP
   Sr. Vice President, Chief Medical Officer
   Presbyterian Healthcare Services
   2501 Buena Vista Dr. SE
   Albuquerque, NM 87113
   505-923-5609
   hasmar@phs.org

10. Selma Harrison Calmes, MD
    Consultant in Anesthesiology
    Los Angeles County Department of the Coroner

11. Josephine Young, MD, MPH
    Chief Operating Officer
    Pediatric Associates Inc., P.S.
    14711 NE 29th Place Suite #255
    Bellevue, WA 98007
    425-460-5669
    jyoung@peds-associates.com

12. Grace Terrell, MD, MMM, CPE, FACP, FACPE
President/Chief Executive Officer
Cornerstone Health Care P.A.
1701 Westchester Drive
Suite 850
High Point NC 27262
www.cornerstonehealth.com
grace.terrell@cornerstonehealthcare.com
336-802-2402

13. Christine Petersen MD MBA
Principal, The Petersen Group
Christinepetersenmd@cox.net

14. Susan E. Ford, MD, MBA, CPE
Medical Director
Amerigroup Community Care of New Mexico, Inc.
6565 America's Parkway NE Suite 110
Albuquerque, NM 87110
P. 505.875.4378
P. 800.600.4441 (After Hours)
F. 866.920.8358
susan.ford@amerigroup.com
www.amerigroupcorp.com

15. Deborah Hammond, MD
Medical Director
Healthfirst
201 669 0842
deborahell@aol.com

16. Traci Ferguson, MD
Corporate Medical Director
WellCare Health Plans, Inc.
8735 Henderson Road
Tampa, Fl 33634
office phone: 813-206-1284
traci.ferguson@wellcare.com

17. Eugenie Komives, MD
former: Vice President and Senior Medical Director, Healthcare Quality
now: Family Physician, Duke Primary Care, Hillsborough (NC)
Public email:– genie416@gmail.com

18. Elaine Batchlor, MD, MPH
    Chief Executive Officer, Martin Luther King Jr. Community Hospital
    Los Angeles, California
    ebatchlor@gmail.com
    cell: 213-798-0264

20. Ellen Strahlman, MD, MHSc
    Senior Vice President, Office of the CEO
    Global Head, Neglected Tropical Diseases
    GlaxoSmithKline
    mobile: +1 484 680 3792
    ellen.r.strahlman@gsk.com

21. Kathy E. Magliato, MD, MBA, FACS
    Cardiothoracic Surgeon
    Director of Women's Cardiac Services, Saint Johns Health Center,
    Santa Monica, CA
    President, American Heart Association - Greater LA County
    Chief Medical Officer, Cordex Systems LLC
    kathymagliato.com (website)

22. Kelly Z. Sennholz M.D.
    CEO, OSL
    Colorado
    DrSennholz@gmail.com
    303-744-3100
    http://www.linkedin.com/in/drkellysennholz

23. Deborah Shlian, MD, MBA
    CEO, Shlian & Associates
    Boca Raton, Florida
    561-988-8780
    dshlian@earthlink.net

24. Kathleen Goonan, MD
    Associate in Health Policy
    Mongan Institute for Health Policy
    Massachusetts General Hospital/Partners
    Kate@GoonanGPS.com
    (508) 869-2186
    Chief Executive Officer
    Goonan Performance Strategies
    Kate@GoonanGPS.com

25. Bonnie C. Hamilton, MD, FAAP
    President-elect American Medical Women's Association, 2012-13
    Fairfield, California
    bonnie.hamilton@sbcglobal.net

Related Reading

Terrell, Grace M., and Bohn, J.M,. *D 2.0: Physician Leadership for the Information Age*, ACPE Publications, 2012

Collins, Jim and Hansen, Morten T *Great by Choice: Uncertainty, Chaos and Luck-Why Some Thrive Despite them All*, Harvard Business Review Press, 2011

Luntz, Frank *Win: The Key Principles to Take Your Business from Ordinary to Extraordinary*, Hyperion, 2011

Sipe, James W, *Seven Pillars of Servant leadership: Practicing the Wisdom of Leading by Serving*, Paulist Press, 2009

Heifetz, Ronald A.; Linsky, Marty; and Grashow, Alexander *The Practice of Adaptive Leadershi: Tools and Tactics for Changing Your Organization and the World*, Harvard Business Review Press, 2009

Olson, Randy *Don't Be SUCH a Scientist: Talking Substance in an Age of Style*, Island Press, 2009

Godin, Seth, Tribes: *We Need You to Lead Us*, Portfolio Hardcover, 2008

Joiner, William B., and Josephs, Stephen A. *Leadership Agility: 5 Levels of Mastery for Anticipating and Initiating Change*, Jossey-Bass, 2006

Drucker, Peter F. *The Effective Executive: The Definitive Guide to Getting the Right Things Done*, Harper Business, 2006

Marquardt, Michael *Leading with Questions: How Leaders Find the Right Solutions by Knowing What to Ask*, Jossey-Bass, 2005

Boyatzis, Richard E., Mcke, Annie *Primal Leadership: Learning to Lead with Emotional Intelligence*, Harvard Business Review Press, 2004

Evans, Gail *She Wins, You Win: The Most Important Rule Every Businesswoman Needs to Know*, Gotham Books, 2003

Patterson, Kerry; Grenny, Joseph; McMillan, Ron; Switzler, Al *Crucial Conversations: Tools for Talking When Stakes are High*, McGraw-Hill, 2002

Evans, Gail *Play like a Man, Win Like a Woman: What Men Know About Success that Women Need to Learn*, Crown Business, 2001

Hunter, James C. *The Servant: A Simple Story About the True Essence of Leadership*, Prima, 1998

Lombardo, Michael M. and Eichinger, Robert W. *Eighty-Eight Assignments for Development in Place*, CCL Press, 1989

CPSIA information can be obtained at www.ICGtesting.com
Printed in the USA
LVOW062146280213

322201LV00010B/201/P